MANAGING PEOPLE
IN

THE
HEALTH
SERVICE

JANE WEIGHTMAN

INSTITUTE OF PERSONNEL AND DEVELOPMENT

Designed by Paperweight
Typeset by Action Typesetting, Gloucester
Printed in Great Britain by
The Cromwell Press, Wiltshire

British Library Cataloguing in Publication Data

*A catalogue record for this book is available from the
British Library*

ISBN 0-85292-641-3

The views expressed in this book are the author's own, and
may not necessarily reflect those of the IPD.

**INSTITUTE OF PERSONNEL
AND DEVELOPMENT**

IPD House, Camp Road, London SW19 4UX
Tel.: 0181 971 9000   Fax: 0181 263 3333
Registered office as above. Registered Charity No. 1038333.
A company limited by guarantee. Registered in England No. 2931892.

**This book is to be returned on or before
the last date stamped below.**

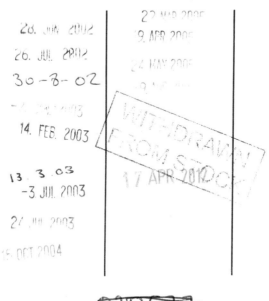

Jane been
at Ul
into
sever
field of mental handicap as a researcher, teacher, lecturer,
and county adviser. She has written widely in a range of journals, and her books on management include *Competencies
in Action* (1994), *Managing Human Resources* (2nd edition,
1993) and, co-authored with Derek Torrington, *Action
Management: The essentials* (1991), all published by the
Institute of Personnel and Development.

£15.95

Dillms

T⁺

MANAGING PEOPLE

IN

THE
HEALTH SERVICE

Jane Weightman BA, MSc, PhD, is a psychologist and has
been associated with the Manchester School of Management
at UMIST since joining in 1980. She has carried out research
into a wide range of management-related topics, including
several in the health service. Previously she worked in the
field of mental handicap as a researcher, teacher, lecturer,
and county adviser. She has written widely in a range of journals, and her books on management include *Competencies
in Action* (1994), *Managing Human Resources* (2nd edition,
1993) and, co-authored with Derek Torrington, *Action
Management: The essentials* (1991), all published by the
Institute of Personnel and Development.

CONTENTS

◻ ◻ ◻

020577

INTRODUCTION

Forty-three members of staff from the hospital were walking 14 miles across the boggy moors in a gentle drizzle. The ones at the front were cheerfully deciding what they were going to eat and drink when they got to the pub. Those at the back were laughing about how damp and miserable they were, because their boots were leaking and the so-called waterproof coats were not living up to their name. Those in the middle were ambling along, talking about various colleagues and work in a gossipy sort of way. At the end of the day everyone said that they had had a great time and felt that the money they had raised towards the scanner had made it all well worth doing.

What had got these people to make such a commitment in terms of time and effort on their day off? Was it the leadership of the organiser? Was it the usefulness of the objective? Was it the fact that it was voluntary? Were people joining friends to do it? Was it the novelty of walking in the moors that appealed to some of them? No doubt there were lots of reasons both generally and individually, but there is no doubt that people working in the health service make extraordinary commitments – and not only by walking the moors – if they feel that something is worth doing and is valued by others.

Managing people in the health service is a complex business, because there are so many more different types of jobs and professions involved than in most organisations. These different competencies need to be co-ordinated to deliver a service to individual patients, each of whom in turn reacts quite differently. But, in the end, the health service really matters to those who work in it and to the patients who receive the care. This complexity of technical expertise, emotions, and individual differences makes the whole business of healthcare fascinating. It also means that managing the people who work in the health service is an important job. To treat people who are often overcommitted as if they were robots will just not work: it is a much more complicated job than such an attitude suggests. Thank goodness that this is so – it would be appalling if we did behave as robots!

This book is intended for people working in the National Health Service and for those working in private health organisations. I have used the word 'healthcare' to refer to people working in either section of the service; and I have used the word 'unit' to refer to the section, department, ward, clinic, directorate, or whatever part of the service and organisation you are responsible for. It is aimed at a variety of people who find themselves, often for the first time, responsible for managing other people on a day-by-day, week-by-week basis. This might include:

❑ nurses in hospitals and the community at ward manager, department manager, or area level

❑ technical specialists with a section to run such as the laboratories, imaging, and instrument sterilisation unit

❑ personnel specialists at the administrative level

❑ doctors taking on clinical directorate responsibilities

❑ GP fundholders and their practice managers

❑ purchasing authority managers

❑ front-line supervisors

❑ people on management courses for the public sector

❑ nursing home matrons

❑ residential care managers.

This is not a book about the strategic responsibility of the personnel department, human resource management, or top management.

I have based my work on well-tried, good personnel practice and established management practice. The rationale for this is that most readers value their own professionalism from their clinical training and also want to see themselves as professionals when managing other people. So to use a professional approach to managing people would be a logical development of their professional expertise. Then again, there are many people who have become wary of the more extreme fashions of managerialism apparent in recent years. I hope my book also tends towards a management style that encourages the development of others rather than just treating them as automata. The emphasis is on management as a job to be done rather than the élitist view of 'being a manager'.

It is intended that this book can also be used in some sense as a personnel primer: when everything else fails, look at this book for a way forward! The emphasis is on *how to do something* rather than lengthy discussions of the issues underlying the particular aspect of managing people. The only exception is Chapter 1, which does examine some of the underlying issues of managing people in the health service.

CHAPTER 1

MANAGING PEOPLE IN THE HEALTH SERVICE

Ivan is a GP in his late forties. This week he has been answering questions at an informal hearing into a complaint made by a patient about the service he gave her. This is the first time a formal complaint has ever been made about Ivan. He has been unable to sleep well for the last six weeks, he has been drinking more alcohol than usual, and has felt very upset by the prospect of appearing at the hearing, even though he feels that the service he offered was reasonable, although not ideal. The biggest surprise was finding himself in this position. The second surprise was the reaction of his colleagues. Many sent messages of support by fax, phone, or letter, or sent him invitations to come round along with offers of solidarity. They were all from people over 40 years old. His colleagues below that age, including two partners, could not understand what the fuss was about: surely this was what you expected in general practice!

Is Ivan's experience a symptom of the changes in the National Health Service (NHS) towards a more litigious approach? Are these changes (if they really exist) typical of other organisations, too? Is it that now everyone is for him- or herself and has less sense of collegiality and co-operation? Do the changes inevitably mean that there will be less commitment by staff to the patients, one another, and the service? Or can we take the changes and still keep that sense of doing something worthwhile and continue to support one another?

1

NHS changes that affect people management

Given that readers of this book will either have experienced the changes in the NHS for themselves over the years or worked only in the current climate, I have no intention of writing a history of the NHS in the 1990s. However, it is worth noting that the following aspects of how the NHS is managed have changed the way we manage staff:

❑ the move away from centralised planning and control
❑ the introduction of a market model of purchaser and provider
❑ local accountability for all aspects of business, including staff
❑ consumer advocacy, such as the Patients Charter
❑ business concepts, such as income generation and joint ventures.

An example of the first listed aspect is the gradual intro-duction of local pay scales. An example of the second is contracts between purchasers and providers listing what will and what will not be paid for. Skill-mix decisions are an example of the third. An example of the fourth is when staff are trained in how to behave towards patients. A (more exten-sive) example of the fifth aspect is the obvious difference between the cultures represented by the traditional NHS and the new approaches when there is large demand for a service. Under NHS management a waiting-list is created, because the resources are seen as limited. However, if extra funding can be found, as it can in the private sector, the hours of operat-ing the service are increased and more staff are employed, so that the need is met without a long waiting-list. The flexi-bility of being able to generate income from the service enables the private operator to commit resources ahead of time, that is take the capital risk, something which the NHS has not been able to do in the past. Some of this flexibility is seen as the main attraction of certain joint projects, such as the MRI (magnetic resonance imaging) scanner at North Manchester Hospital: in this case neither the private nor public sector could justify the full-time use of such a piece of equipment but, between them, they were able to purchase and staff it, making it available to patients at all hours.

All this means major changes in managing people in the health service, both formally and informally.

General changes in culture and management

Alongside revolutionary changes in the NHS there have of course also been major reorientations in the rest of the working world. These have led to various changes in the way staff are managed. In the last few years organisations have increasingly concentrated on such factors as:

❑ being less centralised
❑ handling their staff in a more individualistic way
❑ offering less permanent employment
❑ dealing with rapid changes
❑ managing with fewer layers of managment.

This has been associated with two trends: accountability and empowerment. The trend to measure and make accountable every decision and use of resources is observable in all sorts of management information systems and quality audits, such as ISO 9000. The desire to control everything is understandable, because managers feel under more and more pressure from political masters or shareholders to account for their business. Increasingly people are asked to justify any action, decision, or resource-use with evidence that it is the right thing to do. Again this is understandable if we increasingly see ourselves as becoming a litigious nation and a 'blame culture'. There is a widespread feeling in the health service, for instance, that the public no longer thanks but blames. This is summed up by such remarks as: 'In the past we used to get chocolates and flowers; now we only get the blame if they do not recover.'

However, not everything worth doing is clear-cut. Sometimes we have to act on experienced judgement and trust ourselves to do the right thing and to take a risk – otherwise we shall spend all our time justifying and auditing instead of actually doing things. As someone once said to me: 'No pig got fat by being measured.'

The second trend is the advocation of 'empowered' managers and the development of the people who work for them. One of the main developments in management strategy in the 1990s has been the shortening of lines of communication and command, and the associated attempts to 'empower' line managers. The focus of this has been the individual manager with a department, function, or office to run. Theoretically this manager has been empowered to deliver all that is required, without being dependent on the personnel department or some other specialist function for assistance. In their research on empowerment Hyman and Cunningham (1996) list the traditional people-responsibilities of line managers as:

❑ changing work practice
❑ disciplining subordinates
❑ dealing with absenteeism
❑ dealing with disputes.

This may be compared with their list of the *empowering* responsibilities of line managers, which include:

❑ recruiting people
❑ advising and counselling staff
❑ communicating with staff
❑ conducting appraisals
❑ training staff
❑ leading meetings
❑ communicating upwards
❑ dealing with staff suggestions
❑ ensuring high quality.

Inevitably, a good idea has run ahead of the ability to deliver. At its best, empowerment genuinely allows individuals to develop and to contribute their best work. Yet all too often individual managers feel that they have not been empowered so much as simply burdened with unwanted responsibility – and this without the training, time, resources, or skills to meet their new obligations. Some managers do respond to the new opportunities with enthusiasm and effectiveness; but others are unhappy with their broadened role and begrudge the way that they now have to discharge their people-management responsibilities. I would argue that the empowered line manager needs some initial training and support in how to manage people, and this assumption is the basis of my book.

The new thinking about the role of managers concerns the need to combine traditional skills such as analytical thinking and a financial approach with the ability to listen well, give useful feedback and serve as coach and mentor to staff in order to enhance their satisfaction with, and performance in, the job. By implication all that needs to be done is to develop accountability systems in order to support managers; standards are set, training arranged, feedback on achievements is given, and individual assessment and possible rewards are granted. In this approach the emphasis is on a systematic human resource management (HRM) style to obtain, deploy, and pay the workforce whose performance determines the success of the organisation. For example, the Royal Bank of Scotland (Rick 1996) has established a framework for all HR policies and practices with the idea of creating a high-performing and capable organisation. The Royal Bank of Scotland model includes the following, which are all discussed in this book in more detail:

❑ job and organisation design (see Chapter 7)
❑ selecting for success using a competency-based approach (see Chapter 8)
❑ continuously managing performance using appraisal and coaching as a key responsibility for all managers and supervisors (see Chapter 9)
❑ developing individual capability with individually agreed development plans (see Chapter 11)
❑ business and resource planning (see Chapter 7)
❑ rewarding performance with clear performance standards and rewards (see Chapter 9).

The idea behind these trends in management is to use the best practice of high standards. No doubt they can all be very useful and enhance the effectiveness of any organisation. Unfortunately, they have been used within the cost-cutting environment of many organisations, and so are seen negatively by some, particularly where 'best practice' means 'most competitive' and nothing more. Another irony is that these newer approaches usually mean devolving responsibilities for people to line managers at a time when substantial numbers of these very same managers are facing redundancy. I would argue that the negative overtones of some of the newer ways of managing have a lot to do with the environment into which they have been introduced. The techniques themselves can in reality genuinely improve the organisation of work for all of us.

Strategy, operations, and administration

There are all sorts of different management jobs in any organisation, including healthcare. The basic tasks of management are:

❏ *strategy* – looking to the horizon for what is coming up, deciding what is critical, and making appropriate plans

❏ *operations* – keeping things going day-by-day and dealing with the difference between plan and reality

❏ *administration* – looking after the procedures and policies so the wheel does not have to be reinvented every day.

Different management jobs include these tasks in proportions that themselves differ according to the stages of a career, positions in the hierarchy, and size of organisation. Weightman, Butler, and Griffin (1989) found all of these types of job in a study of management competencies for a health authority (prior to changes).

Strategy

Strategic jobs are often about managing the managers – not the day-by-day stuff but dealing, say, with a major problem that has no 'by the book' answer.

Job-holders tend to have particular areas to promote within an institution and so are involved in promoting change. They are constantly on the lookout for what new trends, demands, or initiatives are coming along that need responding to, implementing, or capitalising on. Jobs of this sort are closely involved with policy-making and getting decisions both made and implemented. People with this sort of job feel that they have the autonomy to get things done. Few are strategic all the time, because most such managers have operations, administrative, or professional work to do. 'Being strategic' means determining the expansion of the service, dealing with outside bodies when the service is questioned, and dealing with competitive tendering. Areas such as discipline, recruitment and selection, and day-by-day budgetary control are often left to other managers. Jobs in this group are about understanding and influencing a wide group of people. Examples of job titles that we met in this kind of work are: assistant unit general manager (out-patients), assistant unit general manager (community nursing services), assistant unit general manager (people with learning difficulties), and deputy unit general manager (patient services).

Operations
Operations jobs are really the other side of the coin from strategic jobs. Operations jobs are about keeping the show on the road, day by day, hour by hour. Their usefulness lies in picking up on the differences between plan and reality. The day-by-day problems need someone to handle them. There are all sorts of uncertainties, such as staff absences, boilers leaking, patients getting confused. All of these need attention quickly and many job-holders in this group see their work as managing people. They are often engaged in recruiting, disciplining, and working out rotas. Additionally they may relieve the stress of those in their sections by being available for a chat, so reducing staff absences and turnover. This form of people management cannot however be divorced from other aspects of operations such as dealing with difficulties, resources, and budgets: if all the emphasis is on managing people there is a danger of losing touch with what really needs doing. It is getting the balance between managing the staff and managing the tasks that is the art of operations jobs.

For people in this group there are principally two people issues. First, there is the tension between how much autonomy to give staff, and the degree of central control. For example, who should decide such things as rotas, resources, patient care, and training? Secondly, there is the question whether the job is seen to be chiefly about nurturing relationships of high trust and consensus, or chiefly about dealing with different groups whose interests conflict. Decisions on these two issues affect the climate of the particular department in terms of how people work together. For example, the members of a high-trust, autonomous group work in a collegial way with one another, whereas those in a centralised group in which conflict has to be managed are more likely to go for formal prescriptions of the work to be done. Whichever style is adopted, these operations job-holders are seen as the main audience for this book. Examples of job titles for this group are: district chiropodist, neighbourhood nurse manager, in-patients services manager, senior nurse-care of the elderly, nurse in charge – elderly day hospital.

Administration

Administration managers need to know the procedures – how a system works and how to get folk to use it. This often involves being able to communicate with various people at various positions in the hierarchy, and being a very good organiser. These jobs are about organisational maintenance, not just the administrative tasks I mention below in the sTAMp classification. It is also about keeping things going by looking after the housekeeping – such things as preparing agendas, writing reports, preparing contracts, attending meetings, and producing minutes would all loom large for people with this type of job. Administration jobs are primarily about systems, procedures, and monitoring – mutually agreed and laid down with other people. These job-holders are not primarily involved in initiating procedures but in putting them into practice. Above all, they need to know the minutiae of the systems they are using. This often involves experience and good contacts with other people to make the systems workable. For example, some of the people we met were responsible for servicing meetings; this required them to know exactly whom to invite, whom to consult over the agenda and minutes, and where the most appropriate venue was for the meetings. But they were not personally involved in the decision-making at these meetings, although they were present. Such job-holders may also find this book useful. In this area we found job titles like health promotions officer, commissioning officer, and personnel officer.

Management analysis: sTAMp

Later chapters of this book have sections entitled 'Questions to ask yourself' but here instead is a device, sTAMp. This stands for 'social, technical, administrative, managerial, and personal' activities. I have used it to analyse people's work where there is some management component. You also could analyse your own work and look at the balance between the three types of work.

❑ *Technical* work is what you do because of your profession, experience, or qualification. It is often done by those working for you and is what you used to do before being promoted. It includes any clinical work you do and your case-load. It also includes using your expertise in giving advice, making policy, doing research, and training others.

❑ *Administrative* work is that which we all have to do to carry out official, authorised duties. It also includes routine activities such as travel, photocopying, and trying to get through on the phone – the sort that 'any literate 16-year-old' could do.

❑ *Managerial* work is where we have the freedom to create precedent. It is about influencing things, nudging things along. Usually it involves not the grand things but those inconspicuous moments when you try to persuade someone to behave slightly differently.

❑ In addition managers have *social* and *personal* activities in a working day – which gives us the phrase 'sTAMp'.

Record how you spend the day by marking whether each activity is mostly s, T, A, M, or p. When I am doing it I call it 'an activity' whenever the subject changes or the person with whom the manager is talking changes. I count meetings as one activity and 'walkabout' as managerial. When I really cannot decide whether an activity is mostly s, T, A, M, or p I score it as a hybrid such as T/M. Table 1 gives some of the advantages and disadvantages of these different types of work.

Questions to ask yourself

What proportion of the day do I spend on what sorts of activity?

Is that distribution acceptable to me?

How does my day compare with the findings for health service workers in the three categories of jobs?

These workers were observed on a day when they did least clinical work. Unlike the people in every other group we have observed, none undertook any personal activities while we observed.

	percentage of time on				
	s	*T*	*A*	*M*	*p*
Strategic people on average	5	4	21	70	0
Operations people on average	6	16	32	46	0
Administration people on average	6	13	55	26	0

Table 1 The balance of work for managers

	Technical	Administrative	Managerial
Advantages	Authority of expertise	Easy to do	React quickly to differences between plan and reality
	Keep in touch with subordinates' work Pride in work	Even pace Keep things running smoothly	Make choices and decisions
	Task-orientated		
Disadvantages	Lose sight of overall aims of organisation Subordinates may be denied scope if technical workload limited 'Generalist' skills not developed	Subordinates irked by demands Comfort of doing something certain creates more administrative work Administrative work can become an end in itself	Hectic pace Building networks can become more important than getting the job done Erratic demands

Particular issues for managing people in the health service

One of the many delights, and frustrations, about working in the health service is that nothing is as straightforward as elsewhere! There is always some extra twist to the managing of people. Here are a few worth considering.

Professionals who accidentally become managers

Most professional people do not choose to become managers but are given responsibility to manage their section. This can lead to individuals' feeling uncommitted to being a manager, unclear about what the role involves, unsure of the management skills required, and unwilling to change. Udall and Hiltrop (1996) use the delightful analogy of leaving the secure island of one's profession to cross this swamp of uncertainty to a new island of expertise.

Managing co-operation in a newly competitive environment

There is a tendency, when markets are new, for a very competitive approach to be taken. This is often because of a misplaced feeling that 'competition' means 'no co-operation'. In fact the reality is that there has to be some co-operation to keep things going. For example, many large commercial organisations belong to local 'salary clubs' where information about terms and conditions are exchanged. Most commercial organisations in established markets try to build co-operative partnerships with their long-term suppliers and customers. This is done by such things as including them in discussions at an early stage, trying to give notice of changes in demand or supply, and dealing with their customers' problems. In the health service this can mean building relationships with particular hospitals, GPs, and suppliers. It can also mean keeping and developing co-operation with neighbouring trusts, clinics, or homes. (Chapter 6 deals with this further.)

Felt fairness

The NHS has traditionally instilled in its members a desire to treat patients fairly and equally at the point of treatment. There is a feeling that the ability to do this is beginning to

11

be eroded by some of the recent changes, such as the existence of fundholding GPs. There has also been a tradition in the NHS of everyone feeling that they have equally poor pay and conditions but that because 'we're all in the same boat it's not so bad.' Yet this sense of equality is beginning to be eroded by quite large differences in pay awards. For example, in 1996 the Government set pay norms, based on review bodies, of 6 per cent for doctors and 2 per cent for nurses. In cash terms this means 6 per cent of a lot compared with 2 per cent of less, which can feel unfair. If these 'felt unfairnesses' are not managed they can begin to undermine morale and consequently commitment to the joint enterprise. Clearly, you as a line manager cannot dispel the felt unfairness described, but you can perhaps try to ensure that not too many are added to the list! For example, 'overmanaging' people when they see others acting with great autonomy can feel unfair, as can the unequal allocation of small privileges at work such as rotas, breaks, and types of work. (See Chapter 4 on 'valuing' for other ideas.)

Managing colleagues in different professions and organisations

To deliver a full service of healthcare we need to co-operate and manage people with different professional qualifications. This can lead to misunderstandings if their orientation is quite different from our own. It can be particularly difficult if managers try to exert control over professionals who resist it. A more productive relationship between professionals and those who manage them is likely if mutual respect and trust is established. This may require some clarifying of values and assumptions. Scholes (1994) suggests that independent-minded, self-motivated, and self-regulating professionals may respect leadership but are often resistant to being managed.

Managing people in the newly privatised sector

For many people moving from a large NHS setting to one of the smaller privatised settings has brought surprises. Some of the terms and conditions of work are very different from those in their previous experience – for better and worse. Some acknowledgement that this transition needs managing

12

helps staff, particularly when a whole group has made the change. This includes the need to deal with the whole change cycle of anger and grief that occurs before individuals are able to cope with the change. It also entails articulating the new setting clearly and frequently in ways that can be understood: not everyone understands management-speak – or indeed wants to.

Managing those who are left
After any period of rapid change in organisations, particularly when there have been redundancies or a lot of people leaving for other reasons, the major management task is to ensure that those who are left do not become too demoralised by the events that have taken place. When those left find themselves doing more and more work but feeling less and less valued they can resent those who left – and those who manage them. (Again, see Chapter 4 on this.)

What is certain that, with all the changes that have taken place in the NHS and in organisations and society generally, most people agree that managing the people well *matters*. I wish you luck!

References

HYMAN J. AND CUNNINGHAM I. (1996) 'Empowerment in organisations: changes in the manager's role,' in *Managers as Developers,* ed. D. Megginson and S. Gibb. Hemel Hempstead, Prentice Hall.

RICK S. (1996) 'Managers as developers or developers as managers?' *in Managers as Developers,* ed. D. Megginson and S. Gibb. Hemel Hempstead, Prentice Hall.

SCHOLES K. (1994) *Strategic Management in Professional Service Organizations (PSOs) – the finders, minders and grinders.* Sheffield, Sheffield Business School.

UDALL S. and HILTROP J. M. (1996) *The Accidental Manager: surviving the transition from professional to manager.* Hemel Hempstead, Prentice Hall.

WEIGHTMAN J., BUTLER L. AND GRIFFIN J. (1989) 'Management Competencies in Tameside and Glossop Health Authority.' Unpublished report.

CHAPTER 2

HOW TO USE THIS BOOK

Generic competencies and personnel expertise

The pick-and-mix model used in this book is based on a study that we (Weightman, Blandamer, and Torrington (1991)), did for the North Western Regional Health Authority. Our 'job composite model' divided the work of personnel specialists into two broad categories: professional expertise relating to some specialised personnel role such as selection or payment; and generic competencies found in several fields of personnel work. I have modified this original model to fit those aspects of managing people that any job-holder responsible for others may need.

The basis of the job composite model is an analysis of the jobs that need doing by people responsible for managing others. Each of these jobs has an associated number of general skills or competencies, such as influencing and advising, that virtually all people who have to manage others need to develop. These are listed below by chapter as the *generic competencies,* and are dealt with in detail in the first part of this book.

Chapter 3 Working in organisations
❑ What makes you credible as a manager?
❑ Using authority and power
❑ Networking
❑ How we influence one another
❑ Negotiating
❑ Understanding organisational culture.

Chapter 4 Working in teams
- ☐ Getting people doing the right thing and getting the right things for people to do
- ☐ Developing leadership and autonomy
- ☐ Valuing: consideration, feedback, delegation, and consultation
- ☐ Teamworking.

Chapter 5 Working with people
- ☐ Working with individual differences
- ☐ Empowering others
- ☐ Counselling and mentoring staff
- ☐ Overcoming stereotypes and prejudice.

Chapter 6 Working with those outside your organisation
- ☐ Communicating with the outside world
- ☐ Facilitating contacts and contracts
- ☐ Turning customers into strategic assets
- ☐ Managing temporary contract staff.

The following list encompasses the main areas of *personnel expertise and competence* that a people manager should have. Every people management job consists of one or more of these roles, some combine two or three; some even have all six. Each role has associated competencies that are described in the second part of this book. The composite is based on facets of professional personnel roles.

Chapter 7 The people manager as human resource planner
- ☐ Getting the right people for the job
- ☐ Matching supply and demand
- ☐ Using HRM approaches
- ☐ Skill-mixing
- ☐ Designing jobs and structures.

Chapter 8 The people manager as selector
- Identifying vacancies
- Recruiting methods
- Different ways of handling the selection process
- Selection decision-making
- Making letters of offer and contracts of employment
- Induction.

Chapter 9 The people manager as performance manager
- Reward and commitment
- Performance management
- Individual performance appraisal
- Managing poor performance
- Discipline and dismissal.

Chapter 10 The people manager as sustainer of staff
- Handling people's responses to change
- Managing change
- Maintaining stability in a period of change
- Coping with stress
- Managing time
- Ensuring health and safety.

Chapter 11 The people manager as developer and trainer
- Deciding what skills to train and develop
- Deciding how to train and develop
- Evaluating training
- Encouraging lifelong learning or personal development.

Chapter 12 The people manager as communicator
- Improving communication
- Using transactional analysis
- Conducting formal interviews
- Communicating with the whole department, section, or team

❏ Communicating effectively in meetings.

The idea of the job composite model is that each individual's job of managing people is a composite of activities drawn from the generic competency and the personnel expertise lists. By looking through the above lists think about your various activities and decide whether:

a) I frequently need to do this
b) I sometimes need to do this
c) I occasionally need to do this
d) I have never needed to do this, but may need to in the foreseeable future
e) I cannot imagine having to do this.

You will thus arrive at a personal profile of desired competencies for managing people in your job. If you then ask yourself whether you have difficulty in any of the *a*)s and *b*)s you should do something about your own development pretty quickly. If you have difficulty with *c*)s and *d*)s you might set them as longer-term development objectives; and any scored *e*) that you have difficulty with you can celebrate, because not having to do them gives you more time for the others! The idea is that different jobs have different profiles and, indeed, different people doing the same job may do them differently and so end up with a different profile, too.

You might therefore choose to read the whole book, only those bits associated with your own profile, or use it as a resource book when everything else fails.

I have throughout used examples and stories from people working in the various health service settings in the UK – they are all true stories, but the names have been changed to protect the innocent! I have also included sequences of *Questions to ask yourself* to encourage you to think about your own practical position. They can also be used to get you thinking and to help if you are facing a problem in a particular area.

References

WEIGHTMAN J., BLANDAMER W. AND TORRINGTON D. (1991) 'Training for personnel specialists in the North Western Regional

Health Authority.' Unpublished but available from NWRHA, 930–932 Birchwood Boulevard, Millennium Park, Birchwood, Warrington, WA3 7DN.

PART I

GENERIC COMPETENCIES FOR MANAGING PEOPLE IN THE HEALTH SERVICE

CHAPTER 3

WORKING IN ORGANISATIONS

Peter is the director responsible for all the non-clinical aspects of a large healthcare trust. This includes estates, catering, laundry, security, and cleaning. A year ago he was responsible solely for estates. When he was offered the new job he asked himself, 'How am I going to work within the organisation with all these new people and areas of expertise about which I know very little?' Should he read books about catering, security, laundry, and so on? Should he try to get to know everyone who works in his area? Should he set out to attend a meeting of staff in each of his sections? Is there some new initiative that everyone needs to be consulted about that would help him to get to know everyone and for them to get to know him? Should he put in an auditing system so that each of the heads of department reports to him weekly? Or would he perhaps do better to concentrate on the things that need doing and assume that the other areas are quite able to maintain themselves until there is some new initiative? These were some of the possibilities for Peter.

There are choices for all of us to make about how we work within an organisation – choices about what we are trying to do and with whom we are trying to do it. These are even more important for managers, because their effectiveness has consequences for their department or section. The resources available to people often depend on the influence of the boss; equally, managers who work well within their organisation get forewarning of major changes and can help prepare staff for them. To demonstrate how important this issue is, just

21

think of the differences between some of the managers you
have worked for in the past!

What makes you credible as a manager?

Like all managers, you are a person with authority stemming
from the position you hold: you are *in* authority, with all the
formal power that that confers. Successful managers have
something more: they are *an* authority, possessing skill,
knowledge, and expertise that others draw on willingly.
'Credibility' is the word used in organisations, particularly
among professionals, to describe this prerequisite for getting
things done. In the growing informality of organisations this
credibility is something that you have to earn and maintain
for yourself. The job title and organisational position help,
but are not sufficient in themselves. Those with high credibility are trustworthy, convincing and respected. They are
listened to and can get things done quickly and with people's
glad co-operation, whereas colleagues who lack credibility
meet resistance and have to rely on the glacier-like speed of
formal mechanisms.

What is credibility? It is the ability to get things done
based on expertise and personal qualities rather than position and power. This means relying on one's own abilities
and on informal ways of getting things done – and done
more quickly and with less fuss. Those who do not have
credibility have to rely on formal procedures and positions
of power. The reluctance of others to comply when there
is no credibility leads to long delays and tedious battles in
implementing change. In our ever more informal organisations the importance of credibility cannot be under-
estimated.

The basis of our credibility is usually an appropriate
expertise and some contribution of such personal qualities
as hard work and enthusiasm. It is a very rare individual
who can rely on personal attributes alone to be credible.
Leadership is more often made up of hard work, understanding of the job, and a position of power. The
components of managerial credibility you might need are:

❑ *keeping in touch with the main task.* It is only by keeping
   in touch with the main task of the organisation as a whole

and the section in which you are located that new ideas can be based on reality. If you lose touch with your operational expertise, you risk losing credibility with your colleagues. Staff may become sceptical about how far you understand current operational problems, and you may retreat further into management and administration. This may in turn create unnecessary systems of control that infuriate staff.

❏ *legitimacy*. Staff on the receiving end of managerial authority respond readily only when they perceive that authority as legitimate. The formal organisational charts, job titles, and pay structures provide *in*-authority legitimacy. Western society and its organisations have developed a taste for informal means to supplement these. Keeping in touch with the main task and maintaining technical competence is the main feature, but *an* authority is also legitimised by such personal characteristics as a willingness to do things and working hard. Belonging to the organisation and showing clear commitment to it can be crucial in being able to influence things. Experience enables some people to develop a 'nose' for appropriate times and actions. They have invaluable legitimacy. The fact that these cannot be learned does not reduce their importance.

❏ *a clear role*. We have found that numerous managerial jobs have no clear role. People with these jobs are not in charge of anything and consequently the individuals, who are often hard-working, experienced, and keen, find work to do. Not all of this is helpful, because it often interferes with other people's work, particularly when the work created is predominately administrative and so increases the amount of administration done by those required to respond.

For further details of these components of credibility, see the series of studies by Weightman (1986) and Torrington and Weightman (1982, 1987, and 1989).

The characteristics that undermine credibility are: appearing to do useless things; adding to the burden of others unnecessarily; and jumping on the bandwagon for personal gain. But different cultures and organisations reflect different things, so your particular organisation may well have other behaviours that add to or subtract from your credibility. The important thing is to know what the basis of your credibility is and to work on maintaining it.

The consequences of not having credibility are that those working for you will be frustrated and less compliant, your peers will take you less seriously, bosses may include you only as a back-up to themselves, and patients, clients, and others outside the organisation may come to devalue the whole organisation.

Equally important in acquiring credibility is the process of maintaining it. There is no use relying on outdated expertise or practical experience gained five or 10 years previously. No young member of staff is impressed by 'Well, we used to do it like this and it worked fine then' or 'Fifteen years ago we had the same problem and I managed to fix it.' It is far better to offer current advice and try to encourage a mutual problem-solving approach.

Questions to ask yourself

Who has real credibility round here?
What is the basis of this credibility?
What is the basis of my credibility?
Is this based on outdated expertise?
What am I doing to maintain my credibility?
Is this based mostly on technical expertise or personal qualities?
What do I do to maintain credibility with my staff?
What do I do to maintain credibility with colleagues elsewhere in the organisation and outside it?
What are we doing to ensure that others can build and develop their own credibility?
Are we doing anything to undermine their credibility?
If so, can we do something about it?

Using authority and power
The previous section used the phrases 'in authority' and 'an

authority'. There is an important distinction between them, because the first phrase implies authority expressed through organisational charts and job titles, control over resources to influence people, whereas the second phrase is based on the personal attributes of credibility to influence people. How this authority and its concomitant power are used to affect behaviour in organisations is an important part of managing people.

The sources of power available to anyone in an organisation are listed in Table 2. Understanding these and using them to change what is decided is part of your responsibility as a manager, because you are being paid to get things done. This does not necessarily mean putting others down, but it does mean maximising the power available to you to influence events appropriately. Examples of using one's power to influence things within a healthcare organisation are: trying to increase the sections' allocation of the budget and so keep extra beds open; increasing the profile of the department so that the service is used more; and trying to get the security staff to help at night with unwanted visitors.

Trying to understand who has power and how it is used also enables you to work better in your organisation, because there is a constant shift of power as new partnerships develop. For example, joint ventures shift power from the traditional hierarchy to those who can effectively influence the partners and represent the home organisation's strategic agenda. Peter, mentioned at the beginning of this chapter, was in this position when there was talk of developing an old psychiatric site as a joint venture with a local house-builder. Similar changes happen when there is a move from central supplies to new supplier–customer partnerships. Instead of carrying out routine administration, the purchasing department has to develop collaborative webs of relationships across departments to negotiate appropriate supplies from a variety of suppliers.

All members of organisations should understand the use of power to influence others – it is not just the prerogative of the mighty. With increased responsibility and accountability at the level of small sections and of individuals we all need to be able to influence what is going on. This is often summed up in the concept of 'empowerment'. Increasingly

Table 2 Sources of power

1. **Position**

   Resources Control access to what others need; whether subordinates, peers or superiors. It includes the following: materials, information, rewards, finance, time, staff, promotion, references.

   Delegation Whether jobs are pushed down the hierarchy; with rights of veto retained or not.

   Gatekeeper Control information, relax or tighten rules, make life difficult or easy depending on loyalty of individuals.

2. **Expertise**

   Skill Being an expert. Having a skill others need or desire.

   Uncertainty Those who have expertise to deal with a crisis become powerful till it is over.

   Indispensable Either through expertise or being an essential part of the administrative process.

3. **Personal qualities**

   Motivation Some seek power more enthusiastically than others.

   Physical prowess Being bigger or stronger than others. Not overtly used in management except as controller of resources. However, statistically, leaders tend to be taller than the led.

   Charisma Very rare indeed. Much discussed in early management literature as part of leadership qualities, but usually control of resources can account for claims of charismatic power.

   Persuasion skills Bargaining and personal skills that enable one to make the most of one's other powers, such as resources.

4. **Political factors**

   Debts Having others under obligation for past favours.

   Control of agenda Coalition and other techniques for managing how the issues are, or are not, presented. Being present when important decisions are taken; control of minutes.

   Dependence Where one side depends on the other for willing co-operation, the power of removal exists. Strikes, or threatening to resign *en bloc*, are two examples.

Source: D. P. Torrington and J. B. Weightman, *The Reality of School Management,* Oxford, Blackwells, 1989.

in organisations there is talk of empowering individuals to take initiatives and responsibility, which ought to include giving the resources to carry out the initiative and having the power to say no. Otherwise it can often feel to staff as if the bosses are just asking them to do more, for less. Those who feel most empowered are those who are confident that they can influence others and get things done.

Questions to ask yourself

> What sources of power do I currently exploit?
> Which others could I exploit?
> Which do I encourage those working with and for me to develop?

Networking

Having a network of contacts both inside and outside your organisation enables you to consult people about new projects effectively. A network also means that we hear when things begin going wrong, rather than having to wait till they actually have gone wrong. Managers who rely on formal relationships are told only what they expect to hear – and only when they have to be told.

Agenda-setting is one way in which people impose their will on the situation around them. The other is by setting up and maintaining a network of contacts through which the agendas are implemented. Agendas and networks are interdependent, because it is often through contact with people in the network that the agenda is kept up to date and appropriate. Networks are quite different from the formal structures (although no substitute for them in large organisations). They are made up of a whole range of people both inside and outside an organisation who can help implement an agenda. They are also a source of information about what should be on the agenda. It is the people who can help things along by speeding things up, providing information, jumping a queue, endorsing a proposal in a meeting, checking data, arranging for you to meet someone with relevant expertise and, of course, doing jobs who all make up a network of contacts. Networks consist of people who work for you, people you have worked with in the past, experts, people who understand the system, and a wide range of personal contacts. Expertise and personal charm are as important as position in the organisation for setting up and maintaining networks. There is usually some reciprocity implied in networks – 'you owe me one' is often heard.

How can we judge whether we are becoming too political in our behaviour? A useful test is to distinguish between setting agendas for action and using networks to implement the agendas. Political behaviour is potentially useful when it is deployed to put agendas into action. It is counterproductive when it is deployed only to build and maintain networks.

'Too much network and not enough agenda' is associated with the type of person who is more concerned with his or her own promotion and position than with getting on with the job. The person who underemphasises networks and concentrates on agendas can be inward-looking and fail to take power seriously; he or she consequently fails to influence events sufficiently. Both these characters can be found in any organisation, but the former is more likely to occupy managerial positions. For example, Ann was the ward manager in a young-disabled unit. She was a friendly, outgoing woman. She willingly went to meetings and conferences, and everyone knew her. Yet her colleagues on the ward felt that she never really had any view of what should happen and so always followed the latest fashions and management requests. In this case Ann would perhaps be better advised to use her obvious social skills for networking to inform her views and develop an agenda about the unit. Another example is Paul, manager of the orthopaedic ward. He is passionate about the needs of people in traction and in hospital for relatively long periods of time. However, his style is rather brusque and intense, so others tend to avoid him whenever possible. He might be advised to learn some of the influencing skills of networking.

Questions to ask yourself

Draw a personal organisational chart showing your formal relations with people within your organisation.
On a second chart, list all the individuals who can affect your performance in your job but with whom you do not have a formal working relationship.

Is there anyone not on my chart who should be?
Are there any people on the chart with whom I need better communication?

How we influence one another

At the heart of working in an organisation is the desire to influence others towards some decision or behaviour that would not otherwise have taken place. The main question is, 'How can we do this when there are so many different personalities involved?' We need to understand how these different people can be understood and influenced. Some of the answer is be found in social science. So a selection of differing models is explored here to demonstrate that we are complex individuals and that we all have a different point of view that needs to be appreciated if we want to influence one another's behaviour.

There are lots of reasons for trying to understand the differences between people. For one thing, doing so helps us to put requests, demands, and expectations to those we work with in a way appropriate to each of them. When we are experiencing difficulties in influencing people it can be helpful to have a range of analytical models for understanding their behaviour and so being able to suggest alternative approaches. When we have a difficult piece of information to impart we can think of different strategies and decide which is most likely to succeed with a particular individual if we have some sort of understanding of that person. Most of us do this instinctively; but the social sciences help us to systematise our thoughts and perhaps suggest new approaches when everything else has failed. Three models of individual differences in behaviour are psychoanalysis, behaviourism, and humanistic psychology. You might well hear people using these terms, so I have included a very brief overview of these three models.

Psychoanalysis

This is based on the view that early childhood experiences influence our adult behaviour. It is still dominated by the work of Sigmund Freud at the beginning of the twentieth century. He concluded that personality consisted of three parts: the ego, superego, and the id. The ego is made up of the individual drives that focus a particular person's nature. It makes people do things differently from those around them and interpret the world differently. The superego is learnt from society and represents the injunctions of parents, schools, bosses, and others about what is acceptable behaviour. The superego can effect the ego. The id is the basic animal instincts that get us going. Freud argues that the personality develops through a series of traumatic stages during which these three aspects come into conflict. Trying to get them into harmony is the business of maturing. (See Freud 1962.)

The usefulness of this model in working in organisations is in understanding that there may be deep-seated reasons for apparently strange behaviours. For example, when you have a member of staff who is constantly upset and angry there may be some unresolved, early experiences that make it difficult for that person to cope with particular current experiences. An offer of counselling to unravel these feelings would be one strategy suggested by the psychoanalysts' point of view.

Behaviourism

Behaviourists argue that we learn through our experiences: it is these that determine who we become. The field is dominated by the work of Burrhus Frederic Skinner. This model emphasises the external control of behaviour. We behave in the way we do because of the history of rewards for our responses. The process of analysing minutely the instructions, tasks, and rewards we have received and manipulating this process to affect behaviour is called 'behaviour modification'.

The usefulness of this model for working in organisations is to understand that one can set up a suitable system of rewards to elicit the behaviour required to run an organisation effectively. Certainly some have tried a systematic analysis of work situations to devise reward schedules and training schedules to modify behaviour. But for most people this feels too manipulative if it is taken too far, and the ethical issues can be very tricky. More common examples are the use of reward management techniques, particularly performance appraisal. This is where we give staff specific objectives, analyse their performance against them, and reward appropriate performance. (See Chapter 9 for further discussion.)

Humanistic psychology
This has been very influential among organisational psychologists. It is really about ideals. It is a description of what could and should be, rather than an analysis of what really is. The emphasis is on becoming an independent, mature adult who can take responsibility for his or her own actions. We can overcome difficulties if we are prepared to take responsibility. Maslow (1954) and his ideas about 'self-actualising' people who work for themselves to see how far their abilities take them is one of the founding fathers of this model. Another is Rogers (1967), who puts the emphasis on adults' being open to experience, living each moment fully, trusting themselves, and becoming responsible for their actions.

The usefulness of this model to working in organisations can be seen in how popular it is among management consultants, with their emphasis on trust, self-development, and empowerment. One particular application has been the concept of stress and the management of stress within organisations. (See Chapter 10.)

There are of course many more models concerned with how we develop such different personalities. The important point for us, however, is the desire to know how we can use these models to influence one another in organisations. As we have seen, there are different perspectives, and we are each likely to have a different way of interpreting others' personalities.

31

So, when we wish to influence someone else we need to consider ourselves, the other person, the interaction that is to take place, and the environment in which it is to take place. Understanding ourselves is important so that we can consider others' reactions to, and expectations of, us; we need to consider the other person in order to take account of his or her experience, personality, and position; then we can think about the nature of the interaction and the suitability of the environment. To influence someone to do something different from what they would otherwise have done it is usually advisable to start with something familiar to, and easily understood by, them. This should be in a relaxing situation.

Questions to ask yourself

Can I think of any behaviours best explained by a Freudian or a behaviourist perspective?
Do I agree with the ideals of humanistic psychologists?
Can I think of someone with whom I work who has a very different style from mine?
Has this person had quite different experiences from me?
How should I try to influence them?

Negotiating

Negotiating is a formal procedure and therefore a special sort of influencing. It may concern negotiating a contract for a service or product. It may concern, equally, negotiating one's own terms and conditions of employment or negotiating with a neighbouring hospital to share a consultant specialist. The important thing is that in most negotiations both sides expect to gain. It is a situation of mutual dependence. Fifty/fifty sharing is a natural solution to the problem in negotiations, because it has an appearance of fairness.

Another sort of negotiation is one in which the number of potential parties on either side increases. In such a case the bargaining power of each member matters less. Here it becomes more useful if interested groups combine forces. So, for example, when purchasers and providers are negotiating on a one-to-one basis it is reasonable to bargain about the fifty/fifty split, whereas if there are several providers and purchasers negotiating together there may be more to say about trying to generate more business than about how exactly it is split. This is certainly a lesson being taken up by conglomerates of GP fundholders, who have found themselves in a stronger negotiating position by grouping.

Questions to ask yourself

With whom do I have to negotiate formally?
Have I done so before, or is this a new relationship?
What do I want out of the negotiation?
What do I imagine the other party wants?
What are my main bargaining-points?

Understanding organisational culture

A special way of analysing organisations, and so being able to work more effectively in them, is to understand organisational culture. It is one of the ways that people use to make organisations more effective and to help manage change. Senior managers are encouraged to try to change the culture, for example from the old 'bureaucratic' NHS to a more 'entrepreneurial' healthcare trust. We are not here concerned with changing whole organisations so, from our point of view, it is probably more useful to see organisational culture as a way of understanding how an organisation works so that when we want to influence events we are not frustrated because we have acted 'counter-culturally'.

Organisational culture is seen as the characteristic spirit and beliefs of an organisation. This is demonstrated, for example, in the conventions about how people treat one another and the type of working relationships that develop. It is cultivated in all sorts of ways and is mostly taken for granted. You really only notice it when you go and work for another organisation and realise that they do things differently. Culture is difficult because it is intangible: you cannot draw it as you would an organisational chart. It is nonetheless felt to be real and powerful. If you unwittingly work against it, you will feel as if you have hit a brick wall.

Four areas to consider are power distance, uncertainty, individualism, and traditional values (see Hofstede 1991):

❏ *Power distance* is that between the least and the most powerful, and the degree of acceptance of it. For example, some hospitals have very formal relations between senior and junior members of staff, so that only the most senior are consulted about changes. Other hospitals use first names and would consult everyone affected by change.

❏ The degree to which *uncertainty* is accepted varies, and affects whether risks are acceptable. For example, departments differ in how much they cross-check results. This then affects how they handle errors.

❏ Differing cultures vary in the degree of *individualism* that is encouraged. We can probably all point to examples of some units in which everyone acts as an individual and to others in which people are very close and present a strong unit identity. Often the style is determined by the nature of the work. For example, research departments relying on dedicated individual insights may accept higher individualism than the ICU (intensive care unit), in which the collective group needs to be closely co-ordinated.

❏ The fourth aspect of culture is the degree to which it is dominated by the *traditionally male values* of rationality, logic, competition, and independence rather than the traditionally female values of intuition and caring. Again there may be differing examples within any one health-care trust, but the overriding culture of senior management may tend towards one rather than the other.

Questions to ask yourself

Have I ever worked in another organisation?
How does my current organisation differ from others in my experience in the way it treats people and influences events?
What would be the best way to get acceptance for a new idea in my place of work?

And finally...

The only purpose for which power can be rightly exercised over any member of a civilised community, against his will, is to prevent harm to others. His own good, either physical or moral, is not sufficient warrant.

J. S. Mill, *On Liberty*, 1859

The graveyards of history are strewn with the corpses of reformers who failed utterly to reform anything, of revolutionaries who failed to win power ... of anti-revolutionaries who failed to prevent a revolution – men and women who failed not only because of the forces arrayed against them but because the pictures in their minds about power and influence were simplistic and inaccurate.

R. A. Dahl, *Power*, 1968

References

FREUD S. (1962) *Two Short Accounts of Psychoanalysis.* Harmondsworth, Penguin Books.

HOFSTEDE G. (1991) *Cultures and Organisations: software of the mind.* London, McGraw-Hill.

MASLOW A.H. 1954 *Motivation and Personality.* New York, Harper and Row.

ROGERS C. R. (1967) *On Becoming a Person.* London, Constable.

SKINNER B. F. (1953) *Science and Human Behaviour.* New York, Free Press.

TORRINGTON D. AND WEIGHTMAN J. (1982) 'Technical atrophy in middle management.' *Journal of General Management,* Vol. 7 No. 4, pp5–17.

TORRINGTON D. AND WEIGHTMAN. J. (1987) 'The analysis of management work.' *Training and Management Development Methods,* Vol. 1, pp27–33.

TORRINGTON D AND WEIGHTMAN J. (1989) *The Reality of School Management.* Oxford, Blackwells.

WEIGHTMAN J. (1986) 'Middle management: dinosaur or dynamo?' PhD thesis, UMIST.

CHAPTER 4

WORKING IN TEAMS

Margaret is busy in the new surgery. She is taking phone calls from patients making appointments to see the GP and from various laboratories and services with results from tests done on patients. She is also trying to organise the patients' records for this afternoon's surgery for the doctor. Helen, the typist, comes in, asking whether Margaret can understand the writing of one of the psychologists. Seeing that Margaret is busy and that the phones are ringing, Helen starts answering the phone and taking appointments for patients. When the local X-ray department phones she passes them to Margaret. How have these two become such an efficient team? Is it their natural style or has something encouraged them to do so? Is it because there is obviously no one else around or is it because they feel that the service they provide is valued? Has the process of moving the surgery from the old building round the corner two weeks ago engendered a new sense of cohesion in the whole team? What would be the consequence if Helen and Margaret worked to a minimum contribution?

This chapter is about aspects of managing people that help to make some teams work better than others. There are two aspects in particular that you need to consider for any team. First: is there something for them to do? If so, is it clear what that is, who is going to do it, and how? Is there a consensus about what the task is – and one agreed not only by those within the team but by those outside who may overlap or need to co-ordinate with the team? The second issue that you need to consider is how the people within the team work together. Do they assist one another to get the best out of the team? Are any processes hindering the team? Are there some sorts of task that the team is better at than others?

Getting people doing the right thing and getting the right things for people to do

Getting the team to do the right thing is your first task in managing people. This is true whether it is a permanent team or a temporary one. Getting the task done is why we go to work. The managerial activities of *planning* and *setting objectives* are about deciding the task. It may come from devolved objectives from senior management, imperative orders from government, demands from partners, providers, and purchasers, or may be internally generated from a desire for change. Once the task is decided, we need to decide how to break it up into suitable chunks for individuals to work on. There are both hard and soft approaches to doing this: these are not stark alternatives but two sides of one coin, and most effective managers use a combination of both.

The *hard* approach to getting the right things done is based on the view that, by carefully analysing the work, we should be able to specify exactly how things ought to be done, and so become more efficient. The appeal of this mechanistic approach is, put simply, this: 'If we only spent just a little more time and effort analysing things we would have a perfect system.' Modern-day examples of this are found among some exponents of the quality movement and competencies approach. For example, very detailed BS 5750 or ISO 9000 quality standards can specify the exact nature of the memos to send if there is a complaint. Similarly competency lists have been seen to include such minute detail as 'Smile at the client when he or she first comes to the reception desk.' An example of this approach in nursing is the desire to break down the whole job into its components and then get less skilled (and worse paid), people to do the more menial tasks. The hard approach expects people to comply with a carefully laid-down analysis of what is required.

The hard approach is useful when a high degree of conformity is required, when there is a lot of temporary or unskilled staff, or when there is a major crisis to be dealt with. The disadvantage is that the more prescriptive an approach, the

37

more people work to rule and show no initiative, because it is 'more than my job's worth'.

The *soft* approach tends to put the emphasis on getting the right things for people to do. This includes an appreciation of individual styles and motivations. Here there is a great deal of discussion about 'empowering' people to take control over their own work and to express their views on how things could be done better. The soft approach emphasises the fulfilment of individual talents. It is about developing people over time and allowing them to make different contributions at different stages in their careers. Sometimes the soft approach emphasises individualism and at others the building of teams. But in either case the aim is to encourage individuals to feel that what they are doing is worthwhile and worth making a commitment to. Some of this is expressed in very caring terms, which makes those from the 'hard' approach feel very suspicious. An example is how some nursing homes allow individuals to express their personal service to the residents in a variety of different ways.

The soft approach with its emphasis on autonomy and collegiality, is most appropriate when the full commitment of people in the team is necessary, for example if the situation is novel, and when everyone needs to deliver the service. A case in point is when health visitors in clinics were faced with a new recommendation on the best way to put babies in their beds to prevent cot deaths, but no one knew quite which was the most effective way of communicating this to parents.

There does seem to be a need for bringing both aspects of getting things done together. One example of how this might be done is by trying to systematise elements of the soft approach so that they can be evaluated alongside the traditional 'hard' method. Using the MCI (Management Charter Initiative, which is the NVQ body for management standards) list of competencies as our starting-point, we felt that the different competencies could fall into four distinct groups:

❑ managing activities – getting things done – and the actions required by the business

❑ managing the analysis of information and resources to solve problems and reach well-considered decisions

❑ managing people – dealing with one's own, and other people's, feelings

❑ managing the vision, values, and assumptions that underpin one's organisation – this involves understanding one's own values and expressing them in strategic ways.

We summarised these competencies under each heading (see Figure 1).

The first two groups of competencies might be described as the hard approach to getting the right things done, and the latter two as the soft approach. We found that teams needed all four groups of competencies, and that the more senior a manager was, the more of the second two groups of competencies they needed, although often they still had to supervise competencies in others from the first two groups. In other words we found that, at different job levels, different groups of competencies fade in and out. The important point of this exercise is the emphasis on the need for different competencies within a team, and that both hard *and* soft competencies are required for sustainable, excellent performance. (This work was based upon the Motivational Driver Model developed by Royston Flude.)

The importance of trying to develop both hard and soft competencies within the health service is seen in almost any unit. There are times when we need the analytical, hard, competencies of making the most of the resources available to us. At other times we have to deal with staff and our own feelings, using the soft competencies. It may be that as individuals we take more easily to one group of competencies than the other. If we are to become useful managers we should try to acquire at least a modicum of the whole range.

Whether a hard, soft, or a hybrid approach is taken, the tasks should be divided up between team members. Custom and practice account for the allocations of many of the tasks. Systematising the distribution of tasks, particularly the new (so that everyone has a sensible job), is a main task of the people manager, and is explored further in Part 2 of this book (particularly Chapter 9).

Figure 1 Competency analysis

Managing vision & values	Managing people	Managing information analysis and resources	Managing activities
Values	Feelings	Thought	Actions

• Establish organisational values and culture • Establish strategies to guide the work of the organisation • Develop profit and growth • Inspire people • Ensure customer satisfaction and quality • Establish integrity and ethics • Establish social responsibility • Communicate in an honest, factual, and accurate manner • Maintain professional standards	• Manage self to optimise performance • Maintain effective working relationships • Respond effectively to poor performance in colleagues and team members • Develop teams to improve performance • Develop management teams • Review internal and external operating environments • Working in a multinational environment • Developing the culture • Communicate sensitively • Technical, commercial and/or organisational experience	*Handling information* • Contribute information to support decision-making • Facilitate meetings and group discussion to solve problems and make decisions • Establish information and communication systems *Analysing resources* • Evaluate and improve organisational performance • Support the efficient management of resources • Secure resources for programmes, projects, and plans *Managing structures* • Adapting to change • Contribute to the provision and development of required personnel • Lead the work of a team to achieve organisational objectives • Manage the human resource component of key projects • Communicate clearly • Technical skills, knowledge, and understanding	• Maintain activities to meet quality requirements • Maintain activities to meet customer requirements • Implement quality assurance systems • Implement change and improvements in organisational activities • Communicate information • Technical skills

Questions to ask yourself

Do we specify what needs doing?
Do we do so using any of the following:
   job descriptions
   procedure manuals
   professional standards
   local standards
   discussion
   annual objective-setting at appraisal?
How far is anyone allowed to decide how to do something?
Would we be upset if they did it very differently from how
we do it?

Developing leadership and autonomy

Having decided the task and how it may be broken down into
appropriate jobs, the second issue you face is how team
members work together. How can they assist one another to
work better? How can you as the manager of a team lead it?

'Leadership' is one of the holy grails of management
writing and talking. Everyone would like to claim it as a
personal attribute, but it is very difficult to get any consensus on quite what it means. It is usually thought to include
the ability to get people to do different things from those that
they would have done, and to do these different things with
some degree of commitment and enthusiasm. Surprisingly it
is quite easy to get people to obey orders at work without the
manager's using any particular skill or personal charm.
However, if we want something more from the performance
of duties than a minimum contribution then something else
is required. A popular distinction between leaders is that
made by Burns (1978), among others, who distinguishes
between transactional and transformational leaders.

❑ *Transactional* leaders use styles of communication and
techniques to clarify task requirements and ensure that
there are appropriate rewards.

❑ *Transformational* leaders are those who articulate a
mission and create and maintain a positive image in
followers and superiors.

41

The latter sort of leader has become the more accepted definition of what 'leadership' is about.

Nowadays you will hear phrases about leadership competencies such as:

❑ Maintain the trust and support of colleagues and team members.

❑ Set up collaborative and consultative working arrangements.

❑ Provide the environment for people to excel.

❑ Nurture individual development.

❑ Recognise success.

❑ Encourage enthusiasm through teamwork.

None of us would disagree with these as worthy ambitions for leaders; they are called 'motherhood terms', in that you can no more be *against* the above phrases any more than you can be *against* motherhood. But it is quite difficult to see how exactly a team leader should go about achieving them. Nonetheless, it seems that the two essential tasks of leadership lie in clarifying the tasks to be done, and establishing suitable enthusiasm and expertise in people to undertake those tasks effectively.

The rest of this chapter is about possible ways that you, as the person responsible for a team, might go about creating an environment in which team members can contribute better to the work in hand.

Questions to ask yourself

Have I worked for anyone who seemed a good leader? Whom have I worked for who was not a good leader? What characteristics distinguish the one from the other? Could I use any of these characteristics to lead others more successfully?

Valuing

If you are to manage staff so that they willingly contribute their efforts and commitment, then there has to be something in it for them. Clearly, salary and the level of interest of the work are important parts of this. But where extraordinary commitment is given there is usually something more. This may be because the work itself is seen to matter; the unusually effective leadership of the manager; or because the individual member of staff feels especially valued.

Most organisations – not just the health service – are suffering from 'innovation overload'. This often happens just when staff morale is lowered because of redundancies and a general levelling of staff differentials. Staff respond to this in different ways. Some do so by withholding commitment. (See Scase and Goffee (1989) on how middle managers remove their commitment.) Some withdraw from extra work. Some increase their militancy. Some simply bow their heads and resolve to work harder – again – like Boxer the horse in George Orwell's *Animal Farm*.

So what can you as a line manager do about it? It is not usually possible to reduce the innovation overload. But, maybe, there is something that could be done about morale. There are several ways that people can help improve the morale of their team by valuing one another. Valuing is a complex social interaction: it has something to do with valuing them as a person as well as the job that he or she does. Four types of valuing are: consideration, feedback, delegation, and consultation.

❏ *Consideration.* People tend to feel a lack of consideration from others when the organisational culture is one of keeping to oneself rather than talking to colleagues. Even at the simplest level such things as eye contact in corridors, saying good morning, smiling, and the everyday courtesies of the working day can make a difference. Evidence from research we have done in a variety of organisations suggests that most people would welcome more of these small gestures at work. Lack of consideration may be one of Hertzberg's dissatisfiers (see Chapter 5).

43

❏ *Feedback.* All too often the enormous contribution and exhausting effort that people put into their jobs seem to lack any perceptible output. People need feedback from their colleagues. This can be in the form of the formal performance appraisal dealt with in Chapter 9. It can also be informal – taking an interest in what everyone is doing. It is not hierarchy-bound: a junior who says 'That's great! How do you do it?' can be very pleasing.

❏ *Delegation.* Members of staff are valued when responsibility is delegated to them, but this should involve delegating *real* responsibility – not just giving people odd jobs to do. Individuals must be trusted to make decisions about what, whether, and how to do things, and not just asked to complete tasks. Otherwise they are likely to work to rule and feel like machines. Responsibility cannot be delegated and then taken away without devaluing confidence and future effectiveness.

❏ *Consultation.* Due to innovation overload it is difficult to create the conditions in which people respond to change with enthusiasm. However, if they are to respond with commitment rather than stoical compliance, then some sort of participation in at least the 'how', even if not the 'what', helps. Although it takes longer to get a decision if you involve more people, they are at least then committed to trying to make it work if they have been involved in the decision process. If you do not include people in the decision process it will take much longer to persuade them afterwards, and they will often use all their creative powers to prove it cannot be done!

Questions to ask yourself

When delegating work to people, do I:
   let them decide whether to do it or not?
   let them decide what to do or not?
   let them decide how to do it or not?
Which decisions do I alone take because it saves time?
Which decisions would I involve my team in making?

Teamworking

Another source of ideas about how to manage people in teams is provided by research studies on groups by psychologists and sociologists that have achieved classic status in the social science and management literature. They are useful to know, because they can provide pointers, warnings or confirmation of our common sense when thinking about how to improve our team.

Group cohesion

Tuckman (1965) suggests that there are various stages that small groups go through before they are mature enough in their relations to be able to work together consistently. These stages are set out in Table 3. They are helpful in showing that group development takes time to become effective, time that varies according to how long the group is going to work together. It may take several months for a long-term group, because the degree of commitment required from each member is high and the risk of personal failure so great, whereas in the short-term, part-time group the risk is lower and the tolerance higher. So when your work team is going through an argumentative period you might wish to ponder whether this is just a stage in developing group cohesion or is down to some other reason. Another time to use this model is when setting up a new group, when you can expect some variation in the emotional climate of the group.

Group interaction

Bales (1950) found that effective groups needed people who helped get things done, that is they were concerned with the 'what' – the content or task facing the group. They also needed people who were concerned about the 'how' – the process, or social and emotional side of working in groups. Team members who were task-oriented were the most influential; those who were interested in the positive, social, emotional aspects were the most liked. Figure 2 summarises his categories of behaviours: behaviours from A, B, and C can all help to make a group work better, whereas D-type behaviours can be destructive. The important thing to remember is that groups (or teams) need both task- and process-orientated behaviours to be effective. Although one's own

45

Table 3 Stages in the growth of group cohesion and performance

Stage of development	Process	Outcome
1. Forming	There is anxiety, dependence on leader; testing to find out the nature of the situation and what behaviour is acceptable.	Members find out what the task is, what the rules are, and what methods are appropriate.
2 Storming	Conflict between sub-groups, rebellion against leader; opionions are polarized; resistance to control by group.	Emotional resistance to demands of task.
3 Norming	Development of group cohesion; norms emerge; resistance is overcome and conflicts patched up; mutual support and sense of group identity emerge.	Open exchange of views and feelings; co-operation develops.
4 Performing	Interpersonal problems are resolved; interpersonal structure becomes the means of getting things done; roles are flexible and functional.	Solutions to problems emerge; there are constructive attempts to complete tasks, and energy is now available for effective work.

Source: Based on B. W. Tuckman, 'Development sequences in small groups', *Psychological Bulletin,* 63, 1965, pp. 384–99.

Figure 2 Bales' interaction process categories

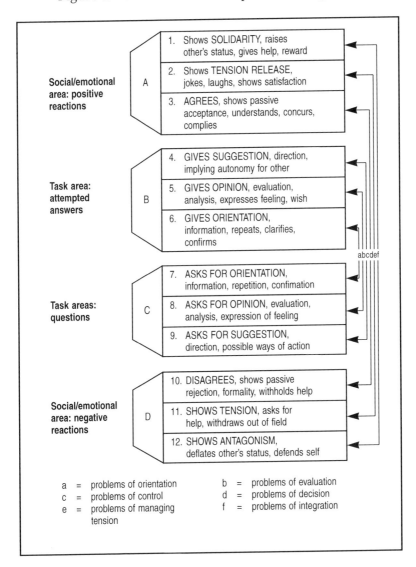

Social/emotional area: positive reactions — A
1. Shows SOLIDARITY, raises other's status, gives help, reward
2. Shows TENSION RELEASE, jokes, laughs, shows satisfaction
3. AGREES, shows passive acceptance, understands, concurs, complies

Task area: attempted answers — B
4. GIVES SUGGESTION, direction, implying autonomy for other
5. GIVES OPINION, evaluation, analysis, expresses feeling, wish
6. GIVES ORIENTATION, information, repeats, clarifies, confirms

abcdef

Task areas: questions — C
7. ASKS FOR ORIENTATION, information, repetition, confimation
8. ASKS FOR OPINION, evaluation, analysis, expression of feeling
9. ASKS FOR SUGGESTION, direction, possible ways of action

Social/emotional area: negative reactions — D
10. DISAGREES, shows passive rejection, formality, withholds help
11. SHOWS TENSION, asks for help, withdraws out of field
12. SHOWS ANTAGONISM, deflates other's status, defends self

a = problems of orientation   b = problems of evaluation
c = problems of control   d = problems of decision
e = problems of managing   f = problems of integration
    tension

Source: Based on R. F. Bales, *Interaction process analysis*, Reading, Mass., Addison-Wesley, 1950.

47

preference may be for particular sorts of behaviour it is as
well to be tolerant of A-, B- and C-type contributions.
Someone (including oneself) who exhibits D-type behaviours
might be encouraged to change by having either the aims of
the group or learning strategies for effective team membership restated.

Team roles

Belbin (1981) developed the work of Bales to look at the
different roles necessary for management teams. He identified eight:

- the *company worker*, who keeps the organisation's interests to the fore

- the *chair*, who ensures that all views are heard and who
  keeps things moving

- the *shaper*, who influences by argument and by following
  particular topics

- the *ideas person* or *plant*, who contributes novel suggestions

- the *resource investigator*, who evaluates whether contributions are practical and finds out where and how to
  obtain resources

- the *monitor/evaluator*, who assesses how valid contributions are

- the *teamworker*, who maintains the group by joking and
  agreeing

- the *completer/finisher*, who tries to get things done and
  suggests conclusions.

At different times each of these roles needs filling for teams
to work effectively. Most of us fill more than one. Again, the
main use of this model is to emphasise that different contributions are required to keep things moving in a group.

Group norms

These are the expectations or implicit rules that are developed within teams to define what is acceptable behaviour
and what is not. Just think back to when you were new in a
job, particularly if you were an experienced worker, to realise

how important these group norms are. Newcomers are expected to comply with the norms as they go through the socialising process of learning the expected behaviours. Eventually the norms become the newcomers' own and are internalised, or they are rejected and the newcomer remains outside the group.

There are two main norms: task norms, and maintenance norms. The first kind influence the way in which the group achieves its goals; what is considered a fair day's work for a fair day's pay varies considerably from one group to another. Maintenance norms develop within the team to help keep it together, for instance regarding style of speaking, little games that are played and cliquey behaviour that distinguishes your work group from your colleagues'. There are also group norms about defining relations with others, such as the boss or other departments.

Questions to ask yourself

Using Tuckman's sequence, where do I think my team fits?
Next time you are in a meeting use Bales's or Belbin's list to check the behaviours of your colleagues.
What are the group norms for my team?
Who has helped to form them?
Do I have little rituals at work associated with say, coffee-breaks or Fridays?
Do a role analysis of your own job. This involves asking all the people who come into contact with you what they expect of someone doing that job. It is not an assessment of how you do it, but what they would expect. It can be quite revealing to realise just what a range of views there are and how they may conflict, be simpler than you thought, or even precisely what you thought!

And finally...

Here are some quotations from business managers about clinical directorate teams. I heard them when working within a particular healthcare trust in which each directorate's management team was made up of a clinical director (a

49

doctor), a care manager (a nurse), a business manager, and an administrator.

'[It is important to ensure] everyone has a say in a proposal.'

'The clinical director will come and chat to me on an informal basis.'

'[Work roles are] becoming more of an equal relationship ... [we are] working towards this.'

'An equal acknowledgement of each other's views is essential.'

References

BALES R. F. (1950) *Interaction Process Analysis.* Reading, Mass., Addison Wesley.

BELBIN R. M. (1981) *Management Teams: Why they succeed or fail.* London, Heinemann.

BURNS J. M. (1978) *Leadership.* New York, Harper and Row.

SCASE R. AND GOFFEE R. (1989) *Reluctant Managers: Their work and lifestyles.* London, Unwin Hyman.

TUCKMAN B. W. (1965) 'Development sequences in small groups.' *Psychological Bulletin,* 63, pp384–99.

CHAPTER 5

WORKING WITH PEOPLE

Sid was the care and business manager in the theatre and high-dependency directorate. He was responsible for ensuring that the operating theatres and the intensive care, high-dependency, and day wards worked efficiently. These were spread over two sites; three miles apart. Every morning he visited each of the theatres before operating began and then visited the wards. Sid had been part of the hospital as a nurse for 20 years; his wife and daughter both worked there as well. This daily 'walkabout' involved talking to many of the surgeons and anaesthetists about equipment, rotas, developments, and budgets. It also involved talking to nursing staff about problems they were having with getting sufficient experienced staff to cover for a series of maternity leaves and sickness. Sid also spent time, on the day I shadowed him, with the technicians in the intensive care ward over the introduction of a new piece of equipment. As Sid went round he joked with people, heard their personal stories, and made notes of things he needed to look into further. By 10:30am he had covered a lot of ground both physically and mentally. His notebook was full of jottings made on his tour.

So what were the strengths of this walkabout? Because he was there every morning before surgery started, everyone knew that they could pass on information and requests without having to waste time in meetings or other more formal methods. By being available to everyone, Sid picked up on problems more quickly than he might otherwise have done. By treating everyone as an important individual, regardless of rank, he was liked and trusted. All this meant that Sid was able to make the resources of the directorate stretch just that little bit further, so that everyone had the satisfaction of attending to the patients more efficiently.

A lot of Sid's job was working with people on all sorts of long- and short-term issues. The great strength of his method of doing this was acknowledging individual differences and trying to meet people half-way to get things done. This chapter is therefore about how to work with people at an individual level and how to try to ensure that we get the best work out of one another. Clearly this whole book is about trying to get better work done with other people, but here we look at those aspects of our interaction with others that affect *how* we work together.

Working with individual differences

If we are going to work successfully with a variety of people, we have to come to terms with the fact that there is quite a wide range of people doing the same job. If we were all the same it would be very boring, but it would also be detrimental to the organisation, because there would not be a sufficient width of experience and opinion when we need to solve problems. By understanding and tolerating these differences we are more likely to get a co-operative, productive effort from those we come into contact with. This does not mean that we have to understand and tolerate all behaviour; indeed, that would amount to indifference. So whereas we should try to influence some people to behave differently, we should show some toleration of individual differences, because this is essential if we are to work with other people.

I have included here three concepts to demonstrate how we can analyse the difference between people. Having analysed and understood the differences we might then want to change that person's behaviour at work. By understanding why they behave differently we are more likely to be able to accept the difference, or at least find a convincing way of helping them to change rather than just saying, 'I want you different.' The three concepts to analyse individual differences are: perception, motivation, and alienation from work.

Perception

This is the term used to describe the process of selecting, organising, and interpreting incoming stimuli. We all do it differently and so perceive a different 'real' world. This world is so stable and familiar to us that it seems curious to discuss 'the way we perceive' the world. But this familiarity and stability has more to do with our own mental processes than the actual sensory input, which is constantly changing. Because we organise the incoming message into our stable view of the world, we make it *seem* stable to us. But your stable world is a different one from mine...

There are several reasons why people may perceive the same situation differently:

❑ physical sensitivity – we differ in our visual and auditory acuity

❑ selective attention – we notice some things and not others

❑ categorisation – we fit things into our existing patterns of understanding

❑ limits on our capacity – we can only deal with a limited amount at any one time

❑ the environment – our expectations and the context determine the kind of categorisation we apply

❑ individuality – our attitudes and personality influence what we perceive.

The act of perceiving is a constructive process by which we try to make sense of our environment and make it fit our experience. The real world is different for each of us because we perceive it differently. As a people manager you will undoubtedly be faced by people who perceive things differently from yourself. Sometimes this is because of a different job perspective and access to information; sometimes because of the amount of time and commitment we have given the topic. Resolving such differences is usually achieved by discussion to unravel the basis of the different perceptions.

Motivation

We use the words motivation, wants, needs, and motives freely both at work and elsewhere. We are in reality guessing what motivates people from the way they behave in different circumstances. There seems little doubt that beyond the very basic needs of food, shelter, and safety our wants are culturally determined. How stable these wants are is the subject of much academic debate.

The most famous model of the variation in motivation across time for the same person and between people is that of Maslow (1954) (see Figure 3). He grouped needs into a hierarchy of five stages. The first two he called primary, concerned with our basic physical needs. The next three he termed secondary needs, which come into play only when the primary ones are satisfied; these are more culturally determined. Indeed Maslow points out that once a primary need is satisfied it is no longer a motivator, whereas secondary needs continue to motivate.

Herzberg (1968) developed Maslow's model with particular reference to people at work. He described the lower-order needs as containing the potential to dissatisfy if they are not met but, once they are met, having more of them will not

Figure 3   Maslow's theory of motivation

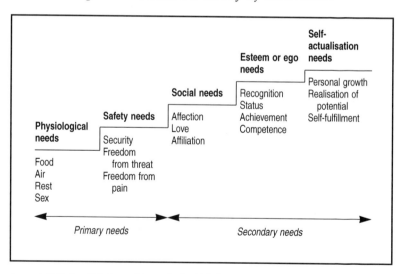

Source: A. H. Maslow, *Motivation and Personality.* New York, Harper and Row, 1954.

increase motivation. These he called the 'hygiene factors': if managers do not get them right there will be complaints and people will be demotivated, but if they are right no one will comment or notice – just like the effect of hygiene in the kitchen. In contrast to the hygiene factors are the 'satisfiers'. People work for these and want more of them. These satisfiers tend to be intrinsic to each person. The list of satisfiers is more culturally determined than the hygiene factors, so your group may have slightly different ones from those listed in Figure 4.

Another view of motivation is given by Vroom and Deci (1974), who discuss the influence on motivation of our expectancy of the success of our actions. The more likely we think it is that we shall be successful, the argument goes, the more effort we shall put in, and vice versa.

Motivating people at work is not just a case of pressing the right button to switch them on. It is about ensuring that they are willing to work, to a set standard, for the rewards offered. This means taking into account individual differences in how they interpret the rewards offered. For example, we all differ in our interests, attitudes, and needs, which in turn affects how we react to different aspects of a job – such as its degree of autonomy, variety and the amount of work to be done. We also react differently to the work environment of our peers, and to the supervision that we receive, and to the organisational climate. In other words, motivating people at work means admitting that different things have different values

Figure 4 Herzberg's theory of motivation

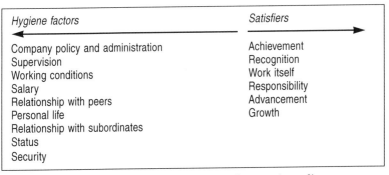

Hygiene factors	Satisfiers
Company policy and administration	Achievement
Supervision	Recognition
Working conditions	Work itself
Salary	Responsibility
Relationship with peers	Advancement
Personal life	Growth
Relationship with subordinates	
Status	
Security	

Source: F. Herzberg, 'One more time: how do you motivate employees?'
Harvard Business Review, January–February 1968.

to different people. This suggests that managers should understand that those who work with them may not have the same orientation to work as they have themselves. As Mills (1956) wrote:

> Work may be a mere source of livelihood, or the most significant part of one's inner life; it may be experienced as expiation, or as an exuberant expression of self; as a bounden duty, or as a development of man's universal nature. Neither love nor hatred of work is inherent in man, or inherent in any given line of work.

Indeed, why some people opt for periphery work and others for core work is an expression of a different set of priorities.

Alienation

It is an ideal world in which everyone is highly motivated and doing exactly what they would choose to do! But there are real dangers if the organisation of work does not give sufficient consideration to the needs of individuals in the organisation. If it is organised so that we are cut off from important decisions, people, and outcomes then we can feel that what we do is alien and oppressive; that is, we are *alienated*. Blauner (1967) argues that alienation consists of four conditions or states: powerlessness, meaninglessness, isolation, and self-estrangement.

❑ *Powerlessness* comes when people feel controlled by others.
❑ *Meaninglessness* is felt when people do not understand the co-ordination or purpose of their work.
❑ *Isolation* is when people do not feel they belong.
❑ *Self-estrangement* is when we do not feel involved with our work.

All of these can happen to people at all levels in an organisation, and they have been well documented in periods of reorganisation. It can be very difficult to find ways of reorienting staff once they have become alienated. It is therefore worth picking up on the early signs so that something can be done to make them feel more valued. We can attempt to pre-empt these elements of alienation by trying to empower staff, setting reasonable objectives, valuing staff, and engendering commitment. These are all dealt with in this book.

Questions to ask yourself

Can I think of someone I work with who generally perceives things differently from myself?
Which of the six factors (see page 53) do you think largely accounts for this?
Which of Herzberg's hygiene factors are currently causing a problem?
What can we do about it?
What do I need to be able to do to motivate my staff?
How have I introduced the idea of change to my staff?
Do we match individuals adequately for individual characteristics?
Is anyone showing signs of being alienated from his or her work?

Empowering others

If there is one concept from the field of HR that has become popular with senior managers it is 'empowerment'; see for example, Foy (1994). This simply means that employees at all levels are responsible for their own actions and should be given the authority to make decisions about their own work. This is not intended just to make people more satisfied with their work but to enable organisations to respond quickly. The advantages claimed for an empowered workforce are better patient services, flexibility, speed, cross-departmental links, improved morale, and compensation for limited career paths.

Empowerment is about ownership of the problem *and* the solution. True empowerment means employees' having the discretion to take decisions about what they feel it is appropriate to do at the time. This empowerment, presumably, also includes the right to be consulted about the nature of the empowerment proposed – and indeed the power to say no to empowerment.

Typical elements of a system to ensure the success of an empowered workforce, from a management perspective, include:

❏ performance evaluations drawn from a variety of sources
❏ variable rewards, including some group element
❏ toleration of errors
❏ enhanced communication
❏ generalist managers and staff
❏ giving yourself time to develop confidence in one another
❏ sufficient resources to deliver some of the solutions generated.

Empowerment can really happen only when there are sufficient resources to take on any training necessary for individuals. Empowerment procedures are too often initiated as a substitute for sufficient resources to get on with the job.

It is also worth thinking about what is in it for each empowered person. This could include such things as:

❏ a team bonus
❏ increased recognition
❏ security of employment
❏ the satisfaction of developing new talents.

Claims to have empowered staff very often fall well short of these ideals. The difficulties with empowerment from the organisational point of view are a greater potential for chaos, a lack of clarity, breakdown of hierarchical control, and demoralisation of those staff who do not want more responsibility. But without there being something in it for the staff they will feel very put upon, the whole initiative will sink in a flurry of accusations about the latest fashion and fad, and it will just not work. As Hyman and Cunningham (1996) found in their research on empowerment in several UK organisations:

> Empowerment in many cases is little different from earlier prescriptions for job enlargement, or at best job enrichment, where employees can exercise discretion and influence over the execution of their immediate tasks, but the overall parameters within which they operate are in many cases not so flexible.

Questions to ask yourself

Which areas do I feel empowered to take decisions in?
Which areas do I empower others to take decisions in?
Could these areas be extended?
What are the consequences if things go wrong?
Have we got sufficient resources to ensure that there is appropriate training?
Have we got sufficient resources so that we can follow up the initiatives of those empowered?

Counselling and mentoring staff

Working with people often means guiding them and trying to get them to see things in a slightly different way. Sometimes we do this by telling them that this is what needs doing. Sometimes we try to sell the idea to them by demonstrating how much better it would be to do it this new way. A third way is when the outcome is less certain but a problem (or potential problem) has been identified and we need some sort of joint problem-solving. When we are trying to encourage another to take responsibility for this problem-solving we may wish to use the counselling method.

Counselling is not the same as giving advice. It is part of the manager's art to enable other people to develop their skills and effectiveness by helping them to find solutions to problems and develop strengths of their own. The role of the counsellor in a counselling interview is to provide a different perspective in which to try out ideas. Those being counselled need to find their own solutions and exercise their own responsibility. Neither the counsellor nor the counselled knows the 'answer' before the interview begins; it emerges from the process itself.

This process can be effective only if the counsellor is willing to listen. Listening requires more than just allowing the other person to talk. There must be a willingness to believe that the other person has something to say, and you should make sure that you have understood what was said, rather than make assumptions from your own point of view. This requires the counsellor to pay attention to the other person and not be distracted. It needs to be clear that there is plenty of time for the discussion, with no furtive glances at the watch. The meeting needs to be private and free from interruption.

The style, warmth, integrity, and authority of the counsellor are going to be the key to how effective the process is. There are some sequences for counselling that seem to suit several people; one such is shown in Table 4. Counselling is not just about getting someone to feel better, it is also about getting people to *perform* better so that they can contribute effectively to the work process. By finding a genuine solution to a problem, there is a better chance of the solution's being permanent.

Mentoring is a form of coaching that reproduces in a modern organisation the traditional working relationship of skilled worker and apprentice by attaching a new recruit to an established member to induct, guide, coach, and develop the recruit to full competence and performance. Mentoring means:

❑ managing the relationship

❑ encouraging the protégé

❑ nurturing the protégé

❑ teaching the protégé

❑ offering mutual respect

❑ responding to the protégé's needs.

Questions to ask yourself

When would I use a counselling model to discuss something with a member of staff?
Are there other times when it could be used?
How would I ensure a reasonable amount of time and privacy?

Overcoming stereotypes and prejudice

In trying to understand other people, we all instinctively use a short-cut method known as stereotyping. This is an essential aspect of dealing with others but can also be a straitjacket if we do not use it carefully. If you have lost your way in a strange hospital and decide to ask someone for directions, you do not

Table 4 Stages in a counselling interview

1 *Factual interchange* Focus on the facts of the situation first. Ask factual questions and provide factual information, like the doctor asking about the location of the pain and other symptoms, rather than demonstrating dismay. This provides a basis for later analysis.

2 *Opiinion interchange* Open the matter up for discussion by asking for the client's opinions and feelings, but not offering any criticism, or making any decisions. Gradually, the matter becomes better understood by both counsellor and client.

3 *Joint problem-solving* Ask the client to analyse the situation described. The client will receive help from the counsellor in questioning and focus, but it must be the client's own analysis, the counsellor resisting the temptation to produce answers.

4 *Decision-making* The counsellor helps to generate alternative lines of action for the client to consider, and then both share in deciding what to do. Only the client can behave differently, but the counsellor may be able to help a change in behaviour through facilitation.

Source: D. Torrington and J. Weightman, *Action Management,* London, Institute of Personnel Management, 1991.

stop the first person you see: you pick out someone from the surrounding crowd who looks like a potential source of good information. You probably pick on someone not in a hurry, neither too young nor too old, with an intelligent and sympathetic appearance. You have, in other words, a working stereotype of who would be an appropriate person to ask. At work we carry round a series of stereotypes that influences all our dealings with other people.

There is seldom time in working situations to abandon all stereotyping. As a way of approaching matters, especially in emergencies, some sort of working hypothesis is needed immediately. The danger of stereotyping is, of course, that people are not treated as individuals but as categories. This is unfair to them, and indeed can be unlawful. It also limits the ability of someone who is overdependent on stereotypes to work with others to the full extent of their abilities. A special form of this is the 'halo effect' of some aspect of behaviour, one which overrides behaviour elsewhere — for example, the care assistant who is always on time but does poor work is seen as an admirable member of staff. Stereotyping often occurs between departments in organisations; so, for example, the laboratory staff are seen as earnest, harassed, and socially ill at ease, whereas the physiotherapists are seen as fun-loving and lively.

Prejudice is where stereotyping is taken to an extreme form, that is when we see whole groups of people as conforming to prejudged behaviours. Some prejudices can be illegal, and in any case are certainly inappropriate in the workplace.

Changing our stereotypes and prejudices is not easy. Changing other people's stereotypes and prejudices is even more difficult, but we need to try, where this is appropriate. Bringing things out into the open is certainly a help. The PC (politically correct) movement, despite some of its absurdities, has been helpful in allowing us to do this. The usual advice for improving our ability to perceive others accurately, and therefore with less prejudice, can be expressed in the following way:

❑ The better we know ourselves the easier it is to see others accurately. A lot of the transactional analysis and assertion workshops are about 'knowing oneself'. For others, an intimate discussion and feedback can be useful. Indeed, the best appraisal interviews include this sort of feedback.

❑ One's own character affects what one sees in others. The material in the earlier part of this chapter on how individual differences arise might help us to deal with this.

❑ The accuracy of our perceptions depends on our sensitivity to the difference between people. Trying to develop a sensitivity about people that looks below the superficial differences is the beginning of wisdom and credibility in managing people.

Questions to ask yourself

When I am feeling aggrieved by the way I have been treated, what do I feel has been misunderstood?
How could I do something about this?
Do I have pet sayings about some of my colleagues?
What do I call other departments in the same institution?

And finally...

There are both verbal and nonverbal clues to whether we are behaving in a diffident, assertive, or aggressive style (see Table 5).

Table 5 Our demeanour towards others

Nonverbal and verbal clues		
Diffidence	*Assertion*	*Aggression*
Moving from one foot to another	Firm, comfortable stance	Leaning forward stiffly
Backing away from other person	Orienting towards other person	Moving against other person
Wringing hands	Hands relaxed	Clenched fists
Eyes averted or cast down	Eye contact with other person	Glaring, expressionless eyes
Voice hesitant or apologetic	Voice steady and clear	Voice staccato and overbearing
Tentative statements: 'I wonder/would you mind/maybe ...'	Firm statements: 'I will/I feel/I know/I want'	Threats: 'I'm warning you/ you'd better'
Negative statements: 'It doesn't matter/ never mind'	Emphatic statements: 'What do you think/ can you help?'	Critical statements: 'This won't do/It's not good enough'
Fillers: 'You know/er/well now/ right'	Co-operative words: 'Let's/what can we do/ how can we?'	Sarcasm: 'You've got to be joking/ what makes you think ...'

References

BLAUNER R. (1967) *Alienation and Freedom: The factory worker and his industry.* Chicago, MI, University of Chicago Press.

FOY N. (1994) *Empowering People at Work.* Aldershot, Gower.

HERZBERG F. (1968) 'One more time: how do you motivate employees?' *Harvard Business Review,* January–February.

HYMAN J. AND CUNNINGHAM I. (1996) 'Empowerment in organisations: changes in the manager's role' in *Managers as Developers,* D. Megginson and S. Gibb (eds.) Hemel Hempstead, Prentice Hall.

MASLOW A. H. (1954) *Motivation and Personality.* New York, Harper and Row.

MILLS C. W. (1956) *White Collar: The American middle classes.* New York, OUP.

VROOM V. AND DECI E. (1974) *Management and Motivation.* London, Penguin Books.

CHAPTER 6

WORKING WITH THOSE OUTSIDE YOUR ORGANISATION

Rachel is a psychologist. She has spent the last 20 years specialising in people with severe learning difficulties. She has always worked in the NHS, seeing individuals to work out programmes of development, and training nursing staff who work with patients on long-stay wards for those with severe learning difficulties. The last few years have been quite different. With the change in responsibility to community care by local authorities and the private provision of homes for people with such disabilities, Rachel now spends most of her time working with people outside the NHS. Rachel still works for the NHS, but most of her patients are now resident outside the hospital.

How should Rachel's behaviour change? Should she carry on giving the same advice and training, or does she need to take a more fundamental review of her role as expert and wait for others to ask? Should she develop contracts to provide expert advice with each of the homes or with the different local authorities? Can they go elsewhere for this advice? To what extent should she monitor the effectiveness with which learning-plans are being delivered, or is that someone else's responsibility?

There has always been a lot of interaction between people working in the NHS and people in local authorities, services, suppliers, and the community, to say nothing of the national and international contacts of many specialist staff. The difference is that many people in the NHS have had to interact with people outside the organisation far more in the last few years than in the past. What has changed dramatically is the style of this interaction. Previously a lot was based on custom and practice and a general sense of working for the public good. Now these relationships have become more formal, with contracts and competition entering the relationship. Not everyone has found this change attractive, but one benefit has been to draw attention to the importance of these outside relationships – relationships that may often have been taken for granted.

We have also had a period of change in quite what we mean by 'the organisation.' In the past, people identified with the NHS and with their particular place of work. Now 'the organ- isation' can mean the NHS, a healthcare trust, a surgery, or a particular specialised, independently funded unit within a hospital, as well as the more obvious meaning of a private institution. No matter what exactly our organisation is, those who are skilled at establishing and maintaining good working relationships with a variety of people and organisations may be increasingly appreciated as this competence comes to be seen as invaluable.

Communicating with the outside world

Many jobs in the health service require people to communi- cate with a large number of different individuals and organisations outside their own organisation. See Figure 5 for examples.

Usually communication is informal – on the phone, face to face – or through routine, formal meetings and letters. However, sometimes one has something more elaborate to communicate, and it is worth taking some time to think about it. There are several questions to do with the nature of this communication that should be answered – not least the need in an ever better-informed world, to meet higher and higher expectations now that accurate and easily accessible infor- mation is available.

The first question you should consider is, 'What do we want to communicate, and to whom?' By clarifying this, the 'how to do so' should be relatively straightforward. We may need to communicate policies, our vision of the future, prac- ticalities, understanding, information, or feelings.

The second question to answer is, 'How do we ensure that our audience is willing?' By being clear about the message

Figure 5 Communication webs

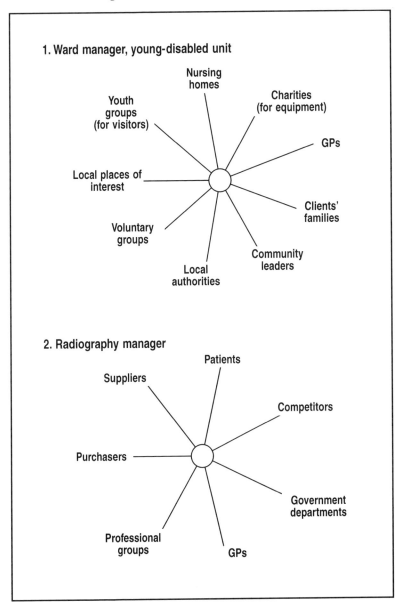

you want others to hear, and by making yourself willing to hear their point of view, the risk of misunderstanding can be reduced. The ideal is always for an honest, frank, and accurate communication to take place between you and others. The reality of life is however that the message is often not clear because of conflicting demands, uncertainty, misunderstanding, and lack of time. It is also the case that promising more than can be delivered is more damaging to a reputation than saying no in the first place; see for example Bourke (1994). Similarly, if the communication is merely dealing with superficial matters and not getting down to dealing with underlying problems, the problems become worse and the reputation of the organisation is destroyed. So the communication needs to be two-way and in touch with the audience of the communication (see also Chapter 12).

The third issue to consider is which style to use. Here it is a case of thinking carefully about who the intended audience for the message is. For example, on September 8 1995, Oxford Radcliffe Hospital produced a 12-page supplement to the local newspaper with the aim of gaining a greater understanding of their work and commitment to it among the local community. The content could have been written from a variety of medical, managerial and technical points of view. However, the presentation was made suitable for a lively local newspaper, written that is in a style accessible to most people in the Oxford area, with an emphasis on the human-interest angle. Some of the same material was also used more formally in various annual reports. So the style was made to suit the different audiences, even though the content was similar.

A fourth issue that is often overlooked is the unintended communications made by an organisation to the outside world. This includes incidental communications and non-verbal impressions. For example, what impact is the organisation having on the local environment through emissions from its chimneys? What impression do the unit's grounds make on visitors? What impression are we giving in our job advertisements and recruitment practices to different members of the community? What does this communicate about our attitudes to staff? Do we show the community our real work by allowing people to see what we do and by visitors' commenting? Again there is no point in overpromising on these fronts. But it clearly makes a nonsense of trying to be a considerate organisation and expecting people to regard you with trust and affection if you are harsh with staff and pollute the local community's air. Similarly, people will remember the reality of their visits to you long after they have forgotten any glossy brochure. The advice is to look after the housekeeping as well as the public relations.

Fifthly, you need to decide which medium suits your purpose. Different media have their advantages and disadvantages. It is not the aim of this book to detail professional communication and media services, because others can do it better. But if you have something that you feel is particularly important or sensitive, it may be worth getting professional help about appropriate media, for example by asking your publicity or management services department.

Sixthly, there are hard and soft ways of communicating with people outside your organisation. Hard ways are the formal mechanisms for people to get together. Soft ways are more informal methods of making an impression, and are more varied. Examples are given in Table 6.

Questions to ask yourself

With whom do I frequently communicate outside my organisation?
How effective is this communication?
With whom else is it important that I communicate outside my organisation?
Who from outside is trying to communicate with me?
Is there a better way for this to occur?
What impression does my unit make to the first-time visitor?
Is there anything simple I could do to make it easier for people to find me or to find what they want to know?

Facilitating contacts and contracts

The recent changes in the NHS have meant that many contacts between individuals and organisations have had to become more formal, because contracts of agreement have been drawn up. However, the vast majority of contacts between people and their organisations are still of the infor-

Table 6 Hard and soft communication with those outside your organisation

Hard	Soft
Advertisements	Public relations
Booklets and videos	Jamborees such as fêtes, parties, and social events
Contributing to local committees on green, welfare and social responsibility issues	Behaving in a considerate way on social responsibility issues
Partnership	Accessibility of staff and managers to respond to queries and complaints
Contracts	
Putting those interested on mailing lists for news of changes in legislation, etc.	Attending seminars and conferences
Contributing to local forums such as Training and Enterprise Councils (TECS)	Networking
Chambers of Commerce	
Sitting on regulating bodies	

mal, phone-call sort. In the course of them people ask for an opinion, share information, and gossip on the grapevine. Without this informal contact, everything would frankly be a great deal more difficult to run. So how can we facilitate the contacts?

Many professional bodies, local teaching hospitals, and universities are good sources of professional networking and also useful for updating professional knowledge and skills. The suppliers of drugs and equipment also invest large amounts of resources in trying to stay in contact with health-care workers. Local seminars, conferences, and training sessions help, too.

When a long-term relationship is likely (and necessary) for professional reasons, it is helpful to find the time to meet *face to face* occasionally rather than always doing things by phone or fax. (Sometimes the most useful part of a formal committee meeting, for example, is the minutes immediately before and afterwards, when all sorts of information and feelings are exchanged informally.) This face-to-face meeting

should include the administrative staff as well as the professional, clinical, staff. Meeting face to face enables people to
bring up little points that would seem petty on the phone but
that, over the years, can niggle. It is often these little points
that, if addressed, make for a better service and continuing
relationship. It may, for example, be more useful to a GP
fundholder to receive properly written laboratory reports
after a few days than to receive a fax of unreadable scribbles
immediately. Only by talking face to face will you find this
out, however.

Long-term professional relationships in which there is
some degree of interdependence are increasingly recognised
as *partnerships* in the management literature. People in the
health service have in fact worked in this way for years,
and yet they are at risk of destroying some of these partnerships just as the idea is gaining credibility in the
commercial world! The idea behind partnerships is a recognition that there is some sort of joint enterprise and common
interest in developing a greater degree of trust and commitment than there is in the conventional customer–supplier
(purchaser–provider) model of the commercial world. Each
side of the partnership offers resources of time, effort, and
money to develop new ways of working that enable each
of the partners to fulfil their part of the bargain more easily.
This often requires one side's taking the other into their
confidence about future plans and developments at an early
stage so that they can influence those plans and prepare
their own organisation for the changes. As an example, the
imaging department of a hospital would talk with local users
such as GPs and clinics as well as hospital wards about
planned changes to the equipment and opening hours to
see whether later evening hours would be appropriate and
generate enough business.

Partnerships can be seen as a way of trying to deal with
competition and co-operation. Just because one is working
in a more competitive market-place it does not mean that
there should not be co-operation. That is what all commercial companies who offer a service or make something have
to do. The one exception is the purely competitive market of
trading. Here no goods or services are provided; it is merely
a question of betting on whether the costs of things goes up,

71

and really has very little to recommend it as a model for a healthcare service.

Questions to ask yourself

How far do I network with people outside my organisation?
Do I encourage others to go on seminars, courses, and presentations?
With whom do I have partnerships?
Is there someone else it would be useful to develop a partnership with?
How could I encourage a more co-operative style with my purchasers or providers?

Turning customers into strategic assets

A particular development of this partnership approach to working with outside organisations is the managing of customers as strategic assets. Those of us who work in the public sector find it very difficult to think in terms of customers, but if we think in terms of patients, clients, and those who demand the service on their behalf then many of the current ideas of working with customers can be useful; indeed some such ideas celebrate the long-established partnerships traditional in the health service.

Successful organisations have long held the view that their important assets include knowledgeable and motivated staff, information and learning systems, technological expertise, supply and distribution contracts, and, increasingly, their customers. It is thought that this last aspect, regarding customers as strategic assets, takes place most successfully if the following conditions are present. If for 'customers' you read 'GPs, purchasers, or patients' it begins to be clearer how this new thinking might apply to the health service:

❑ Current customers (such as GPs and purchasers), are relatively stable.

❑ Individual customers (such as patients, GPs and purchasers) can be analysed in terms of their future demands based on their history to date.

❑ Customers (such as patients, GPs and purchasers) can be exchanged when closures and amalgamation take place.

72

❏ Customers are likely to make fewer demands over time (this is the least likely of the conditions to occur in the NHS for most services, but it may occur in specific areas).

Within a healthcare setting these conditions (except the last one) are very likely to be met because most people prefer to use their local GP, clinic, hospital, or other medical service.

Predicting and developing the service to meet the needs of these 'customers' (as represented by GPs and purchasing authorities) can be done in such ways as:

❏ capturing detailed and useful information on a database
❏ communicating with particular patients, GPs, and purchasing authorities
❏ picking up quickly when there are less frequent requests from patients, GPs, and purchasing authorities to see if they are transferring to other providers
❏ organising new services around particular patients, GPs and purchasing authorities.

Much of this could be done at an organisational level as part of the strategic responsibility of senior management. But there is also a need at a much more local level to manage this responsibility, because it is only at the sectional, departmental, or unit level that the precise detail is understood and can be discussed. You cannot leave it all to top management: they simply do not have the expertise in your specialism. You should keep detailed information about the use of the service and analyse it to see whether any trends or changes in use are apparent.

Questions to ask yourself

What information do we collect about the users of our services?
What questions do we ask of this information in terms of variations in the service requested?
Do we notice quickly enough when there is a drop-off or increase in requests for a particular service?
Do we consult the purchasers about how they see things developing in the future?

Managing temporary contract staff

A particular aspect of working with those outside your own organisation concerns working with contract staff. In particular, nursing has always used 'bank' staff to cover for absent colleagues, but organisations at all levels are increasingly using periphery workers to manage the ebb and flow of work and income. Temporary, part-time, and contract staff (periphery staff) need a different sort of managing from full-time permanent staff (core staff).

❏ *Core staff* are full-time, permanent, career staff working mainly in managerial, professional, and skilled technical positions. They are offered relatively secure employment with an expectation of training and development and career moves when appropriate.

❏ *Periphery staff* are part-time/or temporary staff (or both) employed on a contract basis. They have fewer opportunities for training and promotion within the organisation. Some services have become entirely 'periphery' because more and more they are contracted out.

The benefits to an organisation of employing periphery staff include: improved flexibility and productivity, reduced employment costs, increased resources for core tasks (where contracting-out is used), and enhanced job security for core employees. It can also be attractive to individuals such as professionals with a high-earning capacity and scarce skills, and convenient for some others such as parents of school-age children. However, the great majority of people seek the security of core employment. There are also disadvantages in the widespread use of contract staff:

❏ cost – the short-term gains may be offset against longer-term costs if the contractors are employed at premium rates for a long time

❏ quality and reliability – it is more difficult to monitor work and the safety standards of contract staff

❏ employee relations – the contract staff may upset agreements with trade unions and core staff about terms and conditions.

The management issues associated with periphery staff are as follows:

❏ There is a great need for clear instructions and procedures if things are to be done consistently. This is better done as specifying the 'what' that is required rather than the 'how', because the confidence and contribution of people are better when they feel they have some say in what they do.

❏ Whole jobs are better than bits and pieces. Give the temporary or part-time member of staff something to complete rather than assist or help with, no matter how tempting it is to get them to do all the little things that no one else has got around to. This ensures a more committed contribution.

❏ Periphery staff are almost always more detached emotionally from the organisation than core staff. For that reason they may be more willing to fit in with your requirements. (Many do not *want* to be more involved.)

❏ You should ensure that all the housekeeping information is available for periphery staff – such information as when breaks are taken, where the lavatories are, dress standards, health and safety information, and discipline procedures.

❏ No matter how rare and mysterious the skills brought in by periphery staff, those in the core must have sufficient expertise to manage their contribution otherwise the tail will begin to wag the dog, as happened with some of the early computer contracts in the NHS.

❏ There is a need to recognise that the core staff have to help the periphery staff, so this can mean extra work for them.

❏ If senior staff are spending all their time on the periphery staff, those in the core will feel ignored.

❏ Many of the periphery staff work for more than one organisation and can therefore be a useful source of opinions on the reputation of a particular unit. They can also be your best (or worst) PR department!

Questions to ask yourself

How do we ensure that periphery staff know what to do?
Do we give them enough support to feel welcome?
Who looks after their queries?
In which of the following do we include the part-timers, bank
staff, and temporary staff:
  meetings
  staff development
  appraisal procedures
  coffee clubs
  staff outings
  the Christmas do?
When do we use external consultants?
Is this to save time, to benefit from their expertise, or because
we ourselves find it too difficult?
How do we monitor what external experts are doing?

And finally...

Here are some comments from people working in a healthcare trust on how they have to work with different people
and how they market their directorate:

A business manager felt an important part of his job was

> managing relationships with other parts of the organisation
> such as the information, planning, and finance department,
> despite the continuous change of people.

Another business manager spent quite a lot of time

> selling services in terms of cost and quality to GP fund-
> holders.

A ward sister enthusiastically told me

> we are having an open day to show the general public what
> we provide and how we operate.

A care manager said there was no need for publicity or
marketing, because

> we market our directorate through the quality of the work
> we do on a day-to-day basis and the new initiatives we
> undertake.

References

BOURKE K. J. (1994) 'Strengthening customer relationships and building customer service in a major bank', in *Successful Change Strategies: Chief executives in action*, B. Taylor (ed.). Hemel Hempstead, Director Books.

PART II

PERSONNEL EXPERTISE FOR MANAGING PEOPLE IN THE HEALTH SERVICE

CHAPTER 7

THE PEOPLE MANAGER AS HUMAN RESOURCE PLANNER

Danny was the clinical director of the orthopaedic directorate. The healthcare trust had sent out a letter saying that the hours of junior doctors within the Trust had to be reduced to comply with the government directive on doctors' working hours. There were five consultants in the directorate who were all used to having their own firms of juniors and to organising their own weekend rotas. Danny discussed with the consultants at their monthly meeting what they were to do about the new hours. He had already asked the personnel department to generate on the computer the various ways this reduction in hours could be done. This varied from reducing cover at weekends and nights and increasing cover given by the senior doctors to employing extra staff. All the options meant that junior doctors' hours would be reduced and that they would all be guaranteed every other weekend at home. Finally the consultants agreed on a schedule that would meet the trust's legal requirements and the clinical requirements of the directorate. When the junior doctors heard of this plan they were up in arms, because they saw that their income was to be reduced through lack of overtime and unsocial hours payments. They managed to get the professor of orthopaedic surgery in the local university to intervene on their behalf.

What was Danny to do? Carry out the agreed plan? Get backing from on high? Consult the juniors? Take early retirement and carry on his private practice? In the end he had a meeting with the junior doctors and the senior staff of the trust to explain that the new scheme had to be introduced –

and that was that. A year later the professor who had backed the juniors retired and Danny made sure he got to know the new professor better than he had the old one.

This chapter is about the various aspects of planning that try to ensure there is adequate staffing for the work to be done in a given section or department. At the strategic (whole-organisation) level this would be a major aspect of the personnel department and top management's function. There is also an increasing expectation for the line manager to be involved in 'human resource management' (HRM), because it is only at this level that decisions about what is needed can be integrated with the development of the activities or business of the section or department. The department manager is best placed to do all the prior analysis about the workloads, work methods, and practices that affect the number and expertise of staff required.

Getting the right people for the job

The classic approach to these issues has been human resource (HR) planning, in which an attempt is made to see whether there is likely to be a mismatch between the future needs of the organisation and the supply of suitably qualified and experienced staff. There are several aspects to this.

First, it involves *scanning the horizon* to see what likely changes are coming and what the implications for staffing are. This requires looking at the organisation's plans, government action, trends in techniques, and approaches to the relevant healthcare. Any of these might affect the nature of the work to be done in the department and consequently the number and nature of the staff required. For example, the rise of less invasive surgery has led to more day cases and fewer overnight stays, with obvious changes in staffing required on the wards at night. These changes need to be put alongside the *demand for labour* within the organisation due to current practice and future plans for contraction or expansion of the service.

Secondly there is the business of looking at the *supply of labour* within the organisation in terms of the age, experience, qualifications, pay and conditions, and performance of existing staff. The external supply of labour varies depending on changes in the population, competition for workers from other organisations, and the education and training available in order for people to qualify in particular areas.

Thirdly, a comparison is made between the demand and supply of staff. This *forecast* is the basis for planning. Matching supply and demand can be done manually or by computer.

Except for the simplest cases you are advised to consult the personnel department in your organisation, health authority, or the local training and enterprise council (TEC), who should have access to some sophisticated computer-based HR information systems using payroll and personnel information. The figures that are forecast are not absolutely reliable, because they may be influenced by interdepartmental relations, organisational politics, and the empire-building of senior managers. They may also be affected by artificial restraints from top management, as Rothwell (1995: 171) points out. For example, the board may have put a cost limit or a headcount limit on the organisation. This will affect estimates of labour demand. There will also be arguments about how these costs are counted. Does 'labour' include only the salary or the total employment costs? Are heads counted as actual numbers, or as full-time equivalents?

Once you have got your plans and forecast, Bramham (1989: 155) suggests, you have a basis on which to make plans. Some of the areas that you may need to ask questions about and plan for are:

❏ accommodation – do you need more or fewer treatment rooms, desks, etc?

❏ costs – where will you need additional or fewer resources?

❏ culture – how are the changes going to affect the way people interact?

❏ development – will there be different opportunities for staff development?

❏ industrial relations – how will the unions react to the changes?

❏ organisation development – do we need to reorganise and change reporting relationships?

❑ outplacements – will some people need to find new jobs?

❑ promotion – what opportunities for promotion will there be?

❑ productivity – will these changes affect the amount of work each person can sensibly do?

❑ recruitment – what sort of people will we need to recruit?

❑ redundancy – which groups are likely to face redundancy, and how are we going to handle this?

❑ retirement – do we need to change the ages at which retirement is offered?

❑ reward systems – should we change the salary structures?

❑ training and retraining – in which areas do we need to develop new skills?

❑ transfer – should we arrange transfer of staff voluntarily or compulsorily?

❑ working practices – do we need to rethink the way we work?

Decisions and practice about all of these can affect the way in which people at work are used. Decisions about each also affect how much work gets done, how well the work is done, and how many people you need to do it. For example, if you have a section spread across a variety of buildings you are going to need more staff than if you are all in one place together, but there may still be important aspects of the service that require you to be spread out. In other words, managing the service and the people affects the number of people required. It is rather like having the tail wag the dog if the service is driven by the number of people available but, equally, it makes some sense to ensure that the most economical use is made of staff while ensuring the quality of the service. Many of the topics listed above are among those covered in this book; for that reason I have put those topics in the index, so that you can cross-reference them, rather than describe them again here.

Questions to ask yourself

Which of Bramham's list given above are we currently managing?

Is there anything that could usefully be changed?

Have we got enough people for the work we want doing now and in the future?

Have they got the right skills or competencies for the work?

Do we need to consider training our current staff to be able to do some future work?

Is there anything in Bramham's list above that could be changed to improve the quantity and quality of the work done?

Will we have a problem in the future of too few or too many people in this section?

Matching supply and demand

If the supply and demand for staff are at present more or less in balance then there is no real problem. If there is a mismatch between the supply and demand for staff, then various strategies can be used.

If there are *too many staff* you can decrease the number through early retirement, assisted career changes, encouraging people to seek other employment, sending them on secondment, asking them to work part time or do less overtime, or through voluntary or compulsory redundancy. You could also discourage people from committing themselves to the organisation by giving short-term contracts and introducing flexible working. All of these are better done at an organisation-wide level rather than at local department level, because there may be parts of the organisation who are desperate for your staff or who could certainly use them effectively. Never get involved in these procedures without using the specialist services of your personnel department, because there is legislation on unfair dismissal. Alternatively, you can increase the demand for services by offering it to more people and developing new services.

If there are *too few staff* you could use different recruitment methods. You could try to attract people different from those you usually get, advertise in different places, offer assistance in transport or childcare, or improve the terms and conditions of employment. You could also redeploy, train, and promote existing staff. You could encourage your present staff to take on new work through changes to the terms and conditions, changes in management style and communication, promotion, recognition, or training and development. You could also reduce the demand for more staff by redesigning the work, subcontracting it, or offering staff different arrangements in such areas as overtime.

Questions to ask yourself

Are the supply and demand for staff in balance?
Have we got too many staff?
If so, can we reduce the supply or increase the demand?
Have we got too few staff?
If so, can we reduce the demand or increase the supply?

Using HRM approaches

A development of the classic approach to HR planning has been to integrate the need for people with the planning of the objectives of the organisation. This planning is done at a more senior level than that associated with the jobs held by the majority of readers of this book. Once the strategic plan or initiative is decided it will certainly involve line managers' trying to propose ways of putting it into practice. The strategy may include ideas for improving services for patients, reducing staffing costs, improving the quality of care, or innovations of practice and care.

Approaches to such questions can be on a sectional basis as well as organisation-wide. For example, reducing staffing costs could be done by

❑ improving recruitment techniques so that there are better employees and less turnover
❑ reducing absenteeism
❑ using the skills and time of individuals better
❑ rewarding people more effectively
❑ having annual hours rather than paying for overtime.

Any of these might be effective in reducing staffing costs on a unit.

Questions to ask yourself

> Are there any plans in the pipeline for changes in the service we offer?
> Which of the above list for reducing staffing costs are we doing?

Skill-mixing

One strategy used for reducing staffing costs in the NHS has been to change the balance of jobs done by differently qualified staff, that is a change in the 'skill mix' of staff. This has invariably meant getting less-qualified people doing some of the jobs traditionally done by those more qualified, leaving the latter to do the more skilled work for which they are qualified. For example, care assistants are employed to do the more menial tasks of nurses, and paramedic ambulance staff are asked to help out in accident and emergency departments. Clearly this has been aimed at reducing costs in a climate of budget-squeeze.

The advantage of genuine changes in skill mix, besides reducing costs, is that it enhances the position of each of those involved: it upgrades the skill they use on a daily basis and so helps them to take more responsibility. In such cases it releases the better-skilled person to practise what he or she has been trained to do. This is particularly true in places where there has been a long-term slide into making do with too few staff. In these cases, highly paid professionals have often ended up doing tasks for which they are seriously overpaid and for which a properly trained, but less qualified, member of staff could be recruited, releasing the professional for more skilled work.

Skill-mixing can lead to those left as the sole professional feeling isolated and uncertain where to turn for guidance. It can also mean that the remaining highly qualified staff spend more time organising and managing than actually doing what they feel qualified to do. This does not please everybody, of course. Sometimes it appears that 'skill mix' really means 'scale mix', because the driving force has been the desire to reduce the number of people on higher pay scales rather than genuinely to examine the skill mix of the staff in a particular area of work.

Questions to ask yourself

> Are there people doing tasks that could be done safely by someone less qualified?
>
> If these tasks were put together as a 'job', would that job be coherent?
>
> Would the previous job also be coherent and workable?
>
> What changes would be needed in the organising and managing of this work in terms of rotas, communication, and ensuring quality?
>
> How will those more-qualified staff support one another and the new staff?

Designing jobs and structures

If we are going to reorganise departments by changing the skill mix and increasingly use contract staff, it is very important that *someone* knows what work needs doing! The work to be done should be organised into coherent jobs and into a suitable structure for people to communicate and liaise with one another. There are five main steps that need thinking about:

❏ *purpose* – what purpose will the department serve? Does it provide a service to others in the organisation? Does it deal directly with patients? Does it co-ordinate others' activities? Does it serve any other purpose?

❏ *activities* – what activities are needed to fulfil the purpose? What are the essential things to be done? (This need not necessarily mean everything currently being done – it may include new tasks.)

❏ *job design* – how are the activities best grouped into jobs? Which activities are best done by one person because of the expertise or access to others required? Are some jobs best done by everyone, because they keep everyone in touch?

❑ *authority* – what formal authority do job-holders need to have delegated to them?

❑ *connections* – how can the activities of job-holders be connected through information systems and reporting?

The above questions are the starting-points for considering what we ask people to do at work. Having a clear view of the task to be done is important. But there are other issues to be considered. One way is to use the classic model for *analysing organisations*: the seven S's model of Athos and Pascale (1981). The authors maintain that, to succeed, organisations must focus on all seven areas and that these areas must complement one another. The seven areas are:

❑ *strategy* – includes the plan or course of action. It is about allocating scarce resources over time to achieve specified goals

❑ *structure* – the need to decide what type of organisational chart is appropriate, eg decentralised, clinical, or professional

❑ *systems* – includes how we co-ordinate and inform others about our activities, and concerns such things as meeting-formats, reports, and formal communications

❑ *staff* – means ensuring a supply of suitably trained and motivated staff, with the right skill mix

❑ *style* – is about how managers behave in achieving goals that assist rather than hinder

❑ *skills* – concerns the distinctive capabilities of key personnel

❑ *shared values* – these are the guiding concepts of the organisation that make people feel that they belong to it.

Athos and Pascale's work was based on comparing Japanese and US manufacturing companies; they felt that the Americans were devoting less time than the Japanese to the four soft S's – staff, style, skills, and shared values.

Although UK healthcare organisations are in most ways different from manufacturing companies, the same argument can certainly be made that these latter four S's need careful consideration if healthcare organisations are to work. (In fact they are often neglected.) Without attention to some of these softer aspects of organisation, people may feel estranged, uninvolved, aggressive, anxious, and lack commitment. These feelings are summarised by the sociological term *alienation,* described in Chapter 5 but worth re-emphasising here. Seeman (1959) argues that alienation is composed of the following aspects:

- ❏ *powerlessness* – a sense of low control over events
- ❏ *meaninglessness* – a sense of incomprehensibility of personal and social affairs
- ❏ *normlessness* – a lack of deep commitment to socially approved goals
- ❏ *cultural estrangement* – individual rejection of commonly held values
- ❏ *self-estrangement* – when activities are undertaken that are not intrinsically rewarding
- ❏ *social isolation* – feelings of exclusion or rejection are sensed.

This term is rather less used now, because the emphasis in management writing and discussion is on the other side of the same coin: we hear more about job satisfaction, motivation, commitment, and job involvement. However, any worker can only be as motivated, satisfied, and committed as both the job and the individual him- or herself is allowed to be.

If this model of emphasising the softer aspects of management is used, it is then logical that jobs need to be designed so that people have a suitable chunk of work to call their own and that they can liaise with others to contribute to the whole in a meaningful way. The main characteristics that are likely to motivate people in their jobs are:

- ❏ *skill variety* – having a range of competencies needed for the work
- ❏ *task identity* – completing a whole or identifiable piece of work
- ❏ *task significance* – the work needs to have a significant impact on other people

❑ *autonomy* – individuals need a degree of freedom, independence, and discretion in when and how things are done

❑ *job feedback* – the tasks are more easily achieved if the work itself gives direct and clear information about how it has gone

❑ *dealing with others* – how much staff have to deal with other people varies and different amounts suit different people

❑ *friendship opportunities* – establishing informal relationships at work is again of varying importance to different people.

As an example of how these characteristics work, many of these ideas have been incorporated in the concept of patients' having a named nurse: not only does the patient know who their carer is, but the nurses get some of the above characteristics in their working day.

The major ways of redesigning (or designing) jobs are:

❑ *job rotation* – moving from one job to another to reduce boredom and increase skills. For example, in the instrument sterilisation department (ISD) staff are moved round from receiving goods from theatre, to unpacking and putting in the steriliser, to checking instruments are clean, to packing sets up ready for use.

❑ *job enlargement* – increase in the number of tasks done by an individual. An example would be the ambulance paramedics mentioned above on accident and emergency department work.

❑ *job enrichment* – broadening the responsibilities and increasing the autonomy for decision-making. The increased responsibilities of ward managers, and indeed the change of title from 'nurse', is an example.

❑ *autonomous work teams* – the team decides how, when, and for how much the work is done. The idea of clinical directorates is to give autonomy to multidisciplinary teams.

❑ *leadership models* – when the vision of the leader is sufficient to give meaning and significance to everyone, jobs can feel more worthwhile. It is however difficult to achieve this.

❏ *quality movement* – concentration on the process of the work rather than the people. But this assumes people will be challenged by the need for constant improvement.

All of these can be used successfully at section or departmental level. However, they can also feel very manipulative if staff are suspicious, feeling aggrieved over pay and conditions or left feeling uncertain about their future. Like all change, this needs careful managing and implementation.

None of the above will be terribly effective if the department, section, or unit is poorly organised and has poor structures. Table 7 gives a check-list for reviewing the organisation of your unit.

Questions to ask yourself

Can I describe the seven S's for my organisation?
Do they seem compatible?
Does any of us show signs of alienation?
Can anything be done about it by changing some of the soft S's?
What about redesigning the jobs?

(*Look also at the questions in Table 7.*)

And finally...

The following are examples of the need for planning the use of staff from a healthcare trust:

❏ The use of theatres and the need to get a precise costing of them have to be considered. Some consultants are over-running their time in the theatres and so the question is, who pays for the overtime? One way round this has been to get consultants to manage their lists by having whole days rather than half days in the theatre.

❏ The maternity unit was getting regional manpower figures on the future number of midwives needed and the number of projected deliveries. A decision had to be made as to how typical the trust's catchment area was compared with the regional figures.

Table 7   Check-list for reviewing the organisation of your department or section

Step 1 The *purpose* of the department or section
(a) Does it meet a basic business need, like purchasing or providing, or is it intended to make things run more smoothly, like personnel? Is it necessary?
(b) Is it set up on the basis of output, like business objectives to be achieved, or on the basis of inputs, like people and problems? Are the outputs already being produced elsewhere?
(c) Does the department exist to deal with matters that other managers find uninteresting or unattractive? If 'yes', are the reasons good enough?

Step 2 The *activities* to meet the purpose
(a) Does the section bring together those who share a particular skill or those with a particular responsibility?
(b) What activities have to be carried out to meet the purpose?
(c) How many people with what experience and qualifications are needed for those activities?
(d) How many ancillary staff are needed? How can that number be reduced? How can that number be reduced further?
(e) Are all the identified activities needed? Is there any duplication with other sections and departments? Is there a better way?

Step 3 *Grouping* the activities
(a) How much specialisation is needed? How will this specialisation affect job satisfaction, commitment, and efficiency?
(b) Are boundaries between jobs clearly defined and in the right place?
(c) Will job-holders have the amount of discretion needed to be effective?

Step 4 The *authority* of job-holders
(a) Do job titles and other 'labels' indicate satisfactorily what authority the job-holder has?
(b) Do all job-holders have the necessary equipment – like keys, computer codes, and information – for their duties?
(c) Do all job-holders have the required authorisations – like authorisation to sign documents – that are needed?
(d) Is the authority of any job-holder unreasonably restricted?

Step 5 *Connecting* the activities of job-holders
(a) Do job-holders know what they need to know about the activities of their colleagues?
(b) Are there enough meetings of staff, too few, or too many?
(c) Are there enough copies of memoranda circulated for information, too few, or too many?
(d) Are job-holders physically located in relation to one another in a way that assists communication between those who need frequently to exchange information?

❏ A directorate was looking at the workload activities of the staff and at the dependency of individual patients. This was to enable them to plan what sort of staff they needed, and how many.

❏ Another directorate was obtaining information on waiting-lists so that it could draw up plans for various initiatives such as operating at weekends and evenings. This had obvious implications for staffing and who was to pay for it.

❏ Looking at the case mix (including care profiles) allowed one group to manage their resources better – particularly the specialist technical staff required for the assessment stage.

References

ATHOS A. AND PASCALE R. (1981) *The Art of Japanese Management: Applications for American Executives.* New York, Simon and Schuster.

BRAMHAM J. (1989) *Human Resource Planning.* First edition, London, Institute of Personnel Management.

BRAMHAM J. (1994) *Human Resource Planning.* Second edition, London, Institute of Personnel and Development.

ROTHWELL S. (1995) 'Human resource planning' in J. Storey (ed.) *Human Resource Management: A critical text.* London, Routledge.

SEEMAN M. (1959) 'On the meaning of alienation', *American Sociological Review,* Vol. 24 pp783–91.

CHAPTER 8

THE PEOPLE MANAGER AS SELECTOR

Gloria, a grade F nurse, came into the office on Monday to say she was giving in her notice to leave. She had got a job at the neighbouring private hospital which, although it pays the same salary, fits the weekly hours of work into four day shifts rather than five days. This rota suits Gloria rather better, because she is attempting to do a further qualification to improve her basic nursing registration, and the college-based course runs all day Wednesday, which the private hospital can guarantee her off.

If you were her immediate boss, what would you consider the appropriate next step? First, do you want to fight to keep her? This is not usually the case in the NHS, in which there is a tradition of individuals' deciding their own career moves. But things are different in other organisations, where some individual negotiating may go on at this point. Secondly, it is necessary to ensure that all the right procedures for handing in one's notice are complied with and that a suitable acknowledgement of Gloria's service is made. Then comes the task of thinking about whether and how to replace Gloria.

This chapter is about what to do when there appears to be a vacancy. This is usually when an existing staff member leaves but it can also be when there are plans for expanding or changing a service. Very few of us ever have the task of selecting a completely new team from scratch. Most of us experience the selection of people as one-off events. Although the personnel department has tried-and-tested procedures for dealing with this, there are important aspects of the procedure that involve the relevant person's line manager: only the latter can know in detail the work that needs doing. There is also the opportunity to bring in changes, if required. We all expect to meet the staff who will work with us and certainly an interviewee for a job would similarly expect to meet his or her immediate boss before accepting a job.

Identifying vacancies

The business of replacing or recruiting someone is an opportunity to rethink what we want the person in that job to do. Do we want the same work or something different? Do we want to split the job into a different combination with other members of staff? Is this an opportunity to move people around? The process of recruiting and selecting someone is also the point at which strategic ideas of restructuring and change can be put into effect. For example, Oxford Regional Health Authority instituted programmes of cultural change to help units make the transition from being bureaucratic organisations to becoming more entrepreneurial, proactive, and autonomous after the 1991 NHS Act. This involved a competency model of the work of top and senior managers to inform the recruitment, selection, and development of managers (Iles and Forster 1994).

An overall strategy for staffing can frequently lead to the position that, whenever someone leaves a post, senior staff question whether it really needs refilling. In a climate of cost-cutting and reducing staff numbers the strategic question is often received at the operational level as 'How can you justify this post – surely you can manage without them/with someone less qualified or experienced by reorganising and managing more efficiently?' Which, to say the least, can feel very aggravating to tired staff who see a colleague leaving.

Once you have decided that there is a genuine need for recruitment, how do you get started? The personnel approach to selection is to try to be as systematic as possible, and to reduce the costs of selection as far as possible. Traditionally this has meant looking at a systematic description of the tasks required in the job and then specifying the personal attributes of the individual to do these tasks. This rather makes the assumption that the work and the individual will not change very much over the years. One way that some organisations, using a version of personnel management called human resource management (HRM), have tried to overcome the difficulty of predicting future requirements for change in a job is to look at the personal attributes of individuals to see whether they have the potential for change and development. This approach makes the assumption that such attributes are measurable and predictable. Like so many aspects of working with people, there is no perfect system, and each of us prefers a slightly different model of society. What I have given here is the tried-and-tested personnel approach to selection, with some of the more frequently used HRM methods. (A further review of the issues involved in selection is found in Iles and Salaman (1995).)

To get going, your first task is to *work out what you need.* This means specifying the sort of person you might appoint. This might include:

❑ consideration of *longer-term* aspects of the job such as plans for the organisation and section, and the distribution of competencies and ages within the organisation. (These issues are considered in Chapter 7 on planning.)

❑ deciding *what work you want doing* by reviewing the job description or using a competencies approach. Having a vacancy is a good opportunity for introducing change, so it is worth having a good think at this point rather than rushing in to appoint another Gloria, or indeed anything other than another Gloria! This involves analysing what we want done in this particular job now and for the foreseeable future. When drawing up the job specification it is better to use phrases like 'To do ... (and some verb)' rather than 'responsibility for ...' or 'assistance with ...', otherwise the job does not really stand on its own.

The second step is to draw up a *job description.* The conventional way of doing this, well described in ACAS's booklet (1986), is to remember the following points:

❑ the main purpose of the job – expressed in one sentence. If you cannot find a main purpose then the job needs reviewing!

❑ the main tasks of the job - using active verbs like 'cleaning', 'writing', or 'repairing' to describe what is done rather than vague terms such as 'in charge of' or 'deals with'.

❑ the scope of the job – to indicate its importance. This can be done by describing the value of the equipment or materials handled, the degree of precision required, and the number of people supervised.

This format, sometimes called job analysis, is well suited to a competencies approach whereby the statements lead on to descriptions of the behaviours that the job-holder would need to exhibit in order to do the things described.

The third consideration is known as a *person specification.* This is where the knowledge, skills, and abilities of the ideal candidate are drawn up. There are innumerable lists to help you draw up this specification, but the simplest is to think in terms of the technical skills and knowledge that the successful candidate needs in order to do the things in the job description; then think of the interpersonal, generic, competencies needed for someone to be able to function in the job. The important thing is to set an appropriate level for these characteristics. Too high a specification may lead to a lack of a suitable candidate; one too low may underestimate the problems associated with the job.

Fourthly, we need to make decisions about the *terms and conditions* associated with the job. In most instances this is carried out in association with the personnel department, which ensures some comparability across departments and institutions.

In a rational, systematic organisation there would be a logical examination of the real needs of the section for the work to be done, perhaps using some of the methods given above. This would be followed by an assessment of how many people were doing the work, and some decision about whether there was a need for further staffing. However, the whole issue can nowadays become more 'political'. Management in all its various guises has so emphasised the need to cut staff numbers that a backlash is developing of defending jobs. So it is sometimes necessary to point out what would not be done if a post were not refilled or retained. As an example, one organisation I visited had a decision at top level that all posts with 'assistant' or 'deputy' in the title would be abolished. This led to all sorts of ingenious retitling and lists of major responsibilities and tasks that would not be done if the people in these posts were lost. The most astute operators used the stated aims of the institution as the starting-point of their list of tasks that could not be done without the 'assistant' and 'deputies'.

A fifth consideration concerns the *core and periphery* issues, such as whether a full-time, permanent core worker is wanted or a part-time, temporary, periphery member of staff. There are serious management issues associated with these decisions. Many organisations have become very enthusiastic about employing part-time, temporary, or contract staff, because this allows the organisation to have the staff at busy periods with the minimum of financial costs. However, there are other costs: the less commitment one makes to a member of staff, the less he or she makes in return. Also, a periphery member of staff can require more managing and organising, and this burden often falls on those who work alongside the temporary member, because they know where things live, who needs what sort of attention, and all the details of working practice – and they are the ones there when the question is asked. So the managing of periphery staff is often – through default – done by the more junior, permanent, staff. However, a periphery appointment maintains flexibility over future changes in demand or the type of work done.

By this point you should have some idea about the decisions you need to take about whether to recruit, and about what sort of job and person you are looking for.

Questions to ask yourself

Do we need an extra person or can we rearrange the work between existing staff?
What plans do we have for this section?
What work do we want done?
What sort of person would we need to do this sort of work?
Do we want a full-time, permanent, person or a part-time, temporary, appointment?

Recruiting methods

Recruitment is the business of getting sufficient and suitable candidates for the job at a reasonable cost. There are various methods of recruiting people – see Table 8. The best method is the one that produces the most suitable candidate within reasonable cost restraints.

This early stage of the recruitment process requires both the organisation and the individual to send messages to each other so that there is a mutual exchange and negotiation (Herriot 1989). We can probably all remember examples of job advertisements that attracted us to apply and others that were very off-putting. The nature of the recruitment literature does influence who applies for the job, so it deserves careful attention if we want to attract the right sort of people.

Table 8   Methods of recruiting candidates

Internal advertising
Word of mouth
Local schools and colleges
Local newspapers, radio, TV, and cinemas
Jobcentres
Trade unions
Commercial employment agencies
National newspapers
Specialist and professional papers
Recruitment consultants
Headhunters
Recruitment fairs
University appointment boards
The officers association

Using word-of-mouth methods of recruitment are worth considering, such as phoning people you know who might be aware of someone looking to move jobs or return to work. This can often lead to a good fit of personal qualities. It has also been established that people recruited by word of mouth tend to stay longer (Jenkins 1986). However, there is a danger here of basing selection on 'like' recruiting 'like', and ending up with a department of clones. It can also lead to discrimination against those who are not part of the network – and to that extent may even be illegal.

The personnel department usually deals with the administration of recruitment: such things as placing advertisements, sending application forms, and job descriptions to potential candidates, receiving the completed forms, and answering general telephone enquiries. Line managers need to ensure that the personnel department knows of any specialist needs for recruitment to this post. This might include advertising in a particular trade journal well known for job advertisements; for example the *New Scientist* carries a lot of vacancies for research assistants and technicians in the laboratories of hospitals and universities. The advantage of the personnel department's dealing with this administration is that some sort of consistency between departments can exist, promoting a corporate approach for different posts, and that there is actually someone whose job it is to deal with the phone calls and paper work – rather than someone in another department constantly called away from his or her proper work.

Questions to ask yourself

Do we need anything special doing when recruiting for this post?
Does any of us know someone who might be interested and appropriate?

Different ways of handling the selection process

Having recruited a group of candidates who are interested in the job, you now have the task of selecting one of them. The complexity and permanence of the job is reflected in the nature of the selection procedure. For a straightforward job, a simple selection interview usually suffices. For more complex jobs, a variety of selection procedures is used; some of these procedures are listed below. The important thing is always to involve the immediate supervisor in the selection procedure in order to ensure that he or she is committed to welcoming the new worker and that the new worker has the opportunity of assessing whether he or she could work with the supervisor.

Here is a list of some of the most common types of selec-

tion procedures, with some of their advantages and disadvantages:

Application forms

These form the basic information for the initial trawl for
short-listing. They can also form the basic starting-point of
the personnel record. They need to be designed for easy use,
with the opportunity for individuals to add material where
they want. Usually there is a standard, organisation-wide
form for you to use. Check that you are not asking for illegal
information – for example concerning marital status, children, or race.

Assessment centres

This is when a number of short-listed candidates undergo a
range of selection procedures, including group exercises.
Their value lies in the variety of evidence collected, but they
are expensive to run, both in time and money.

Curriculum Vitae or CV

These are similar to application forms, except that candidates
select their own way of presenting data about themselves and
their careers. There are now commercial companies offering
help in the presentation of career experience, emphasising
the competencies demonstrated at work. There are usually
real differences between people; there can also be unreal
differences between them, but there are also often big differences in the quality of their CVs!

Interviewing

Whenever research is done on selection interviews they are
found to be unreliable, and yet most selection processes
include an interview. It is an important part of the initiation
ritual. It is also important for everyone involved in the decision to gather in one place to see how it falls. This aspect of
the ritual is ignored at one's peril! So how to get the best
from the interview?

❏ Preparation – compare the candidates against the job and
   person specifications. What do you need to ask more
   about? Prepare some questions; these should be about

abilities and experience, and be related to the job – not personal questions. What questions are the candidates likely to ask? Can you answer them? Look after the house-keeping: a quiet room, free from interruption, plus someone to greet the candidates and give instructions on how to find you.

❑ Conducting the interview – this is all about the balance between formality and friendliness. Describe to candidates what is going to happen. Start with easy questions, such as what they do in their current job. The flow of the interview is the interviewer's responsibility. To encourage the flow, use questions like 'I was particularly interested in ...'; to discourage the flow, use questions like 'I would prefer it if we could move on to ...' Eye contact and nodding will keep candidates talking; looking at watches and papers will shut them up. It is worth keeping notes openly during the interview. Towards the end, ask candidates if there is anything they would like to know, and try your best to answer them. Tell them when they can hear the outcome of the process and ensure that someone sorts out travel expenses and a tour of the place if this has not already been done.

❑ Immediately afterwards, make notes of your impressions. To what extent do they meet your specification? Has their career pattern shown appropriate development and progress?

Recruitment agencies
These can handle some of the preliminary recruitment and selection process, such as advertisements, application forms, and testing. They are often very useful in recruiting periph-ery staff, and also in specialised fields such as bank nurses and computing, because they maintain contact with indi-viduals over several years. However, the final stage of selection should be retained in-house, except for a very temporary post, because it is important that the individual chosen does 'fit in'.

References

References are frequently used in public-sector employment but are almost unheard of elsewhere. They often tell you more about the writer than the person written about. Their main purpose is to confirm judgements and information formed elsewhere. They should be taken up with the candidate's permission only.

Selection testing

These are tests of attainment and performance related to the skills necessary for the job. It is important that the prescribed test really does test the skills needed, and does so fairly. Selection tests should be selected very carefully, because many are out of date. The use of psychological tests, which look at general intelligence and attitudes, is more controversial. They may be used for young people with no track record, but should always be used only by trained people.

Questions to ask yourself

How much time and effort can we give to this selection?
What might be the consequences of an ill-judged appointment?
Who should be involved in the selection procedure?
How can we match our findings with our specification?

Selection decision-making

Having generated the written evidence about the candidates and, in almost every case conducted interviews, you should now decide whom to offer the post to. Some system of comparing the results with your original criteria should be set up, either formally or informally. The advantage of having a slightly more formal system is that you can defend yourself against possible claims of discrimination more easily than if you have just said something such as, 'I really like her because I think she'll fit in.' This is not to say that you should ignore the informal 'feel' about the suitability of a candidate, but you should be able to demonstrate that your selection decision is reasonable and not prejudiced. One way of doing so is to list on a sheet of paper the main criteria for selection along one side, with the names of the candidates across the top, and tick when you have evidence that they have the competence. Another is to sort candidates into 'possibles' and 'probables', and then have a good look at the probables.

It is obvious to most people that the selection needs to be done fairly. In addition to the social and legal obligations, there are increasing economic and demographic reasons to avoid unfair bias. The areas in which discrimination most commonly occurs are job advertisements, recruitment procedures, and promotion, training, and transfer policies. It is the responsibility of the personnel department to monitor these and to help with specific problems.

One of the two most important legal statutes on gender discrimination is The Equal Pay Act 1970, designed to stop discrimination in terms and conditions between men and women. This is interpreted as 'equal pay for equal worth', and means that the two parties cited in a legal case have to be working for the same employer and at the same establishment. The second important statute in this area is the Sex Discrimination Act 1975, aimed at removing unfair discrimination in non-contractual areas of employment and at indirect discrimination in such things as advertising. This means that you cannot prefer to promote one gender alone, for example by choosing to develop only men or only women; there has to be demonstrably equal access to experience. The Race Relations Act 1976 and the Fair Employment (Northern Ireland) Act 1989 follow very similar lines. The Equal Opportunities Commission and the Commission for Racial Equality are specialist organisations for help on this subject. Your personnel department, health authority, or the local TEC can all help with advice.

The decision-making in selection happens at three main points: first, when drawing up a short-list for interview from the initial application forms and CVs; secondly, when testing and interviewing; and finally, when making the final selection decision. All three stages must comply with the anti-discrimination laws.

Questions to ask yourself

Are we discriminating unfairly?
Do our contracts unintentionally discriminate unfairly against certain applicants?
Is what we are doing legal?

Letters of offer and contracts of employment

Usually the personnel department sends out a formal letter of an offer of employment. If this is accepted they usually deal with all the administration, such as the formal contract of employment, health and safety regulations, pay scales, pensions, and starting dates. Everyone should have a formal contract of employment. Some people choose to send out more informal stuff about the department with this mailing. However, in large establishments this may not be advisable, because the bureaucracy can bog things down. The important thing is to ensure that the selected person knows when, where, and to whom to report on starting.

Questions to ask yourself

Who is responsible for administrating the letter of appointment and contract of employment at my place of work?
Do I want to contact the person before he of she starts work?

Induction

The first few days or weeks of a new job are amazing: remember the mixture of excitement and terror? This needs to be picked up. There may be a formal induction programme or handover period, but there are also informal, housekeeping things to be attended to particularly in a busy workplace. If this is someone's first job then he or she has everything to learn – but at least not very much is expected of him or her. Even an experienced person needs support, because he or she will still not be familiar with basic things about systems and procedures in the new place of work. Make sure that someone is deputed to take the recruit round, to answer any questions, and to take him or her on breaks.

Questions to ask yourself

On what day and at what time are we expecting the new worker?
Have we arranged for someone to be free for a suitable length of time to explain things?
Who will be the new worker's named mentor for the first few weeks?

And finally...

Here are some extracts from job applicants' references. What would you make of them?

Mr Appleby is now coping much better with his problems...

Miss Barrow has not quite fitted in here, but I'm sure that was our fault rather than hers.

Mr Cardiff has set himself very high standards and has complete faith in his ability eventually to reach them.

Mrs Durham has very neat handwriting and excellent time-keeping. (*Mrs Durham is applying for a senior management post in local government.*)

Dr Edgware can be a pain, but if you have a sufficient supply of aspirin the pain is probably worth it.

References

ACAS. (1986) *Recruitment and Selection Advisory Booklet No. 6.* London, Advisory Conciliation and Arbitration Service.

HERRIOT P. (1989) *Recruitment in the 1990s.* London, Institute of Personnel Management.

ILES P. A. AND FORSTER A. (1994) 'Collaborative development centres: the social process model in action?', *International Journal of Selection and Assessment,* Vol. 1 pp59–64.

ILES P. A. AND SALAMAN G. (1995) 'Recruitment, selection and assessment' in J. Storey (ed.) *Human Resource Management: A critical text.* London, Routledge.

JENKINS R. (1986) *Racism and Recruitment: Managers, organizations, and equal opportunities in the labour market.* Cambridge, Cambridge University Press.

CHAPTER 9

THE PEOPLE MANAGER AS PERFORMANCE MANAGER

Phillipa is the clinical nurse specialist for critical care in a large teaching hospital. She has been in the post for a year, having come from another hospital outside the area. She found a hard-working group of 81 nurses and technicians in place – people who in many cases had worked in these wards for as long as 20 years. Most of the nurses are on high grades, reflecting their professional skills. There is a constant flow of new techniques and technology coming on-stream in this department. Phillipa wants to discuss with her staff the changes that they are having to deal with, and prioritise the development of each member. The unit is rather isolated geographically from the rest of the hospital and is, by their own admission, élitist. Phillipa wants to find some way of getting all the staff to work together despite the problems of shifts, nights, part-timers, and professional commitments. She also wants to tackle some of the interpersonal difficulties that arise when there are shortages of staff through illness.

She has considered various approaches: staff meetings, individual talks, informal discussion in her office, and asking the personnel department to do something. In the end she has decided to introduce a developmental appraisal scheme for all the staff, with nurses on G and H grades and the chief technologist responsible for conducting the appraisal interviews. She wants the appraisal scheme to include some objective-setting and discussion of personal development plans (PDPs).

She and I spend two days running an appraisal workshop

for all the senior nurses and technicians; this has been done in two groups because, obviously, the critical care still has to go on despite management training! At the end of the two days an action plan is agreed on how to set up the appraisal interviews. Everyone still claims to feel nervous about the process, but less threatened than before, because they see how such a system can be separated from pay by keeping the reporting forms confidential and 'owned' by the individual rather than the manager, with the staff able to nominate two senior members by whom they would be prepared to be appraised. So far it all seems to be going well.

Managing performance has become one of the buzz-phrases of management. It can mean everything from manipulating pay and other reward systems to ensuring that staff know what they are doing. So a whole variety of claims is made about managing performance. The one certain thing is that nothing quite distinguishes our assumptions about the working relationship so much as our approach to managing performance, that is our assumptions about what is acceptable and what is not. Some would argue for the autonomy of individuals to offer their work in whatever way they feel is appropriate professionally; others want things much more tightly controlled by managers.

Reward and commitment

The way in which people are rewarded is central to the regulation of the employment relationship. Pay arrangements are also central to any changes, including cultural initiatives, because they are the most tangible expression of the working relationship between employer and employee. Managerial perceptions of appropriate pay systems have been subject to considerable change and fluctuation over the years. The basic principles of paying for time or performance are at the heart of any system. Payment for time is relatively straightforward, with determined hourly or weekly rates. Paying for performance is altogether more complicated. The nature of the performance, and whether it is achieved by an individual or a group, has to be considered. Many organisations have ended up with some hybrid system that includes both these factors, as well as all sorts of custom and practice. For example, we (Weightman, Blandamer, and Torrington 1991) found that people in the North Western Regional Health Authority were paid on 2,008 different levels of pay; 78 per cent of these pay points had 10 people or fewer being paid the appropriate set amount. We also found wide ranges for such things as weekly hours, annual holidays, pay for being 'on call', and so on.

It is outside the scope of this book, and is not your responsibility as a line manager, to discuss the advantages and disadvantages of different pay systems; for further information on them see Kessler (1995). However, it is worth noting that the current fashion of 'pay for performance' approaches to managing performance can really only work in an environment in which the staff are given enough discretion in their jobs to be able to affect their actual performance in a significant way; otherwise they will become cynical about the whole initiative. It is also the case that for performance-related pay schemes to make a significant difference to performance about 10 per cent has to be added to the salary bill. In our view this method is currently inappropriate in a health service context.

As a line manager, you are responsible for pay, but this is often merely an administrative task of ensuring that the paperwork associated with hours, overtime, and rotas is up to date and returned before the pay date. Pay administration is a classic Herzberg hygiene factor: if it is OK, no one is troubled, but if there is an administrative error then people can get very upset! However, as a line manager, you are also responsible for engendering commitment from the staff. Rewarding them in other ways than through pay lies within your powers. People work for a variety of reasons, as we saw in Chapters 4 and 5. To gain their commitment you can reward them by valuing their contribution, allowing them autonomy, supporting them through personal crises, and generally treating them as they would wish to be treated. Your personal credibility and leadership will enhance the value of these rewards in the eyes of the staff.

Questions to ask yourself

What does the pay I receive tell me about the organisation I work in?

Do the terms and conditions of the people who work in my section vary?

What about the non-qualified staff?

What about the difference between the conditions of the core and periphery staff?

In what ways do I reward my staff, other than financially?

Performance management

Growing interest in systematic management over the last 10 years has led to the development of 'performance management'. This is usually taken to mean an increased emphasis on specifying what is wanted and rewarding those individuals who are able to deliver it satisfactorily. The normal stages of performance management are:

☐ written and agreed job descriptions, reviewed regularly

☐ objectives for the work group derived from the particular organisation's strategic objectives

☐ individual objectives derived in turn from the above, jointly formulated by appraiser and appraisee. These objectives are results- rather than task-oriented, are tightly defined, and include measures to be assessed; they are designed to stretch the individual and offer potential developmental as well as business needs.

☐ a development plan, devised by the manager and the individual, detailing goals and activities to enable the individual to meet his or her objectives. These could be competency-based; the emphasis is on managerial support and coaching.

☐ an assessment of objectives with ongoing formal reviews, on a regular basis, designed to motivate the appraisee and concentrate on developmental issues

☐ an annual assessment that affects pay, depending on the performance in achieving objectives.

One of the major advantages of performance management is

that managers are forced to give emphasis to formal and planned employee development. Another is that it also enforces a clear role-description and set of objectives agreed by managers and individuals. On the down side, there is a potential conflict between the aim of improving performance, which requires openness and a developmental approach, and the link with pay. This conflict is sometimes resolved by holding separate performance development and performance pay reviews at different times of the year.

Questions to ask yourself

How many of the performance management techniques are being used in my department?
Would it be appropriate to use more?
How would this sit with the desire for some people to be seen as autonomous professionals?

Individual performance appraisal

Performance appraisal is a well-established way of providing milestones, feedback, guidance, and monitoring to staff. A further development, as described above, is to fit this appraisal into a larger and more complete system of performance management. These performance management systems, which are increasingly in use (see, for example, Fletcher 1993), highlight appraisal as a central activity in the good management of staff. The difference from traditional appraisal 'chats' is that the assessment process in performance management tends to be more rigorous and objective, is clearly linked into precise job definitions, is based on organisational objective-setting and individual development plans, and is linked to the pay system.

The essential elements of any performance appraisal are *judgement* and *reporting*. The performance is not being measured simply in terms of the completion of a work rota: it is being judged. It obviously involves discretion, worry about bias, and the possibility of being quite wrong. This judgement not only has to be made but also passed on to other people in such a way that they understand what is intended and take action upon it. Those devising performance appraisal schemes spend most of their energies in finding ways of making the judgements as systematic and the reporting as consistent as possible between different appraisers.

Much of what has been written about the appraisal process concentrates on personal interaction. George (1986) suggests that an effective appraisal scheme is dependent on the style and content of appraisal not conflicting with the culture of the organisation. He suggests that the degree of openness required in the appraisal process is 'unlikely to materialise without an atmosphere of mutual trust and respect – something which is conspicuously lacking in many employing organisations' (George 1986: 32).

Appraisal should therefore reflect the wider values of the organisation in order for it to be properly integrated and to survive in an effective form. The appraisal system can in fact be used positively to display and support the culture and style of the organisation.

The reasons for which you might want to appraise your staff include:

❏ *HR considerations* – to ensure that the abilities and energies of individuals are used effectively. You would hope as a result to know more about the staff and make better use of each individual's talents and expertise.

❏ *training* – it is useful to identify training needs both for new tasks and in order to remedy poor performance amongst your staff.

❏ *promotion* – talking to individuals about their aspirations as well as finding out about their performance assists decision-making about who is ready for promotion.

❏ *planning* – to identify skill shortages and succession needs. If there is a widespread lack of particular skills then some serious planning should take place.

❏ *authority* – the appraisal system sustains the hierarchy of authority by confirming the dependence of staff on those who manage them. It is one of the rituals that underlines who is boss.

The reasons for which staff might wish to be appraised by their managers include:

❏ *performance* – here is an opportunity to discuss what could be done and how one might go about doing it.

❏ *motivation* – talking about the job and the work it involves may remind us why we do it and why we wanted it in the first place.

❏ *career* – bosses can be helpful, because they understand the promotion route well, having travelled the same route themselves.

Many things can impair the judgement, reporting, and effectiveness of the performance appraisal. For example, you should be aware of the following:

❏ prejudice
❏ insufficient knowledge of the individual
❏ the 'halo' effect of general likeability or recent events
❏ the difficulty of distinguishing the performance from the context in which the person works
❏ different perceptions of what appropriate standards are
❏ marking everyone 'just above average'
❏ ignoring the outcome of the appraisal process – for example, if there are no improved resources, training, or changes, then everyone will feel frustrated.

Despite these problems of judgement, reporting, and follow-up, the potential advantages of performance appraisal are so great that the effort is worth expending to make it work.

Most people find the problem-solving approach the most effective form of appraisal interview – when both appraiser and appraisee have the skill and ability to handle the situation. This approach is similar to the counselling interview (see Chapter 5), in which neither party knows the answer before the interview begins. It develops as the interaction takes place. Training in this type of interviewing is widely available. This does not mean that you should do no preparation before the interview. Indeed, quite the contrary. Both parties need to have a good think about the last year's performance, the next year's expectations, and where changes are expected. It is the comparison of your collective views of these that can be the real stuff of a trusting, problem-solving appraisal interview. Experience suggests that the quality of the interview improves as the confidence and trust of the participants develops; so do not expect too much the first time!

Performance appraisal in various guises is now very common; different forms are constantly introduced to try to resolve some of the difficulties listed above. Despite the problems, most people feel that a regular, formal encounter between themselves and their boss is an appropriate (if sometimes disappointing) procedure.

Questions to ask yourself

Is performance appraisal used in my section?
Would it be useful to do so?
Is there some organisation-wide model for me to use?
What do I think would be the main advantages?
What do I think would be the main resistance to the idea?
Where am I going to find the time to do it?

Managing poor performance

One aspect of managing performance is managing the poor performer. We can all perform badly at times. Usually there is some toleration of this, but when it persists something has to be done about it for the sake of the patients, other colleagues, and the individual concerned. Avoiding the issue of managing poor performance does not mean that it goes away. Problems with people at work can be short or long term. For example, most of us are not very good when we have a cold. But there are others who never seem to perform well. It is these individuals with a long-term performance problem that I want to discuss.

Before anything can be done to improve poor performance it is important to establish that there really is a *gap between the required and the actual performance.* Required performance can be communicated to individuals in several ways, for example through:

❑ contracts of employment with an outline of duties
❑ formal rulebooks

- ❏ job descriptions
- ❏ training manuals
- ❏ lists of standards
- ❏ procedures
- ❏ briefing meetings
- ❏ training sessions
- ❏ meetings
- ❏ individual conversations
- ❏ professional training and monitoring.

There may be reasons for an individual's having difficulties with any of these. For example, the written requirements may be poorly thought out, inappropriate, or out of date. Any one of them may be poorly communicated.

When we need information about the actual performance it can be collected in several ways, for example from:

- ❏ personal files
- ❏ timesheets
- ❏ sickness and absence records
- ❏ record cards
- ❏ patients' complaints
- ❏ inaccurate work
- ❏ mistakes
- ❏ colleagues
- ❏ comparison with other people's work
- ❏ unfinished work.

After looking at what is expected and what has actually been done, the question is whether the gap between the two requires attention.

If a gap is established, the next task is to find the *reason for the gap*. Only by finding this can we begin to do something about it.

There are three main types of reason for poor performance. First, there are personal reasons arising from the individual's domestic circumstances, which are of course outside the organisation's control. The main issue is how long and to what extent we allow personal problems to interfere with work. Secondly, there are reasons to do with poor management and organisation. Thirdly, there are individual reasons arising from an individual's not fitting in with the organisation. These reasons are summarised in Table 9.

Having established a gap in performance and found the reasons for it, we are in a better position to do the main job of management – *doing something about it.* Establishing

Table 9 Reasons for problem performance

Personal characteristics
- Intellectual ability inappropriate, owing to poor selection or changes
- Inappropriate robustness or sensitivity due to poor selection or changes in the job
- Poor physical ability, which may change with age or job changes
- Health problems
- Domestic circumstances, such as childcare, parents, or partner
- Family breakup

Organisational characteristics
- Assignment and job impossible to do or understand
- Lack of suitable planning in touch with reality
- Job changes do not make sense to the individual
- Pay felt to be too low or poorly administered
- Poor investment in equipment
- Inadequate training
- Inappropriate levels of discipline, either too excessive or too lenient
- Poor management – either an individual poor manager or a poor management system
- Physical conditions distract from the performance if they are irritating
- Location and transport problems when relocated

Individual characteristics
- Group dynamics being such that someone does not fit in and is made to not fit in
- Personality clash (usually in reality one of the other reasons here, but we all feel this clash occasionally)
- Sense of fair play abused when different views on the right way to do or say things are ignored
- Conflict of religious or moral values
- Inappropriate levels of confidence – either over- or underconfident
- Poor motivation, although usually this is really a symptom of some of the other reasons here
- Poor understanding of the job, despite everyone's efforts to explain

some reasons for the gap gives us a starting-point for dealing with it. Some ways of dealing with it are given in Table 10. Whatever the starting-point, there is a need to discuss the problem performance with the individual concerned; the counselling interview technique discussed in Chapter 5 is appropriate here.

Questions to ask yourself

Have I ever really dealt with the poor performance of one of my staff or do I just hope it will clear itself up?
Try using the process outlined above to analyse the problem next time you are frustrated by a colleague to see whether you can come up with some reason for his or her poor performance.

Table 10 Ways of dealing with the poor performer

The following are not given in order of execution but as starting-points to assist thinking when a problem arises.

Goal-setting. Jointly agree specific, reasonable goals and a date for reviewing the performance.

Training. Make sure that you give appropriate training, preferably on the job, so that there is no problem in making the connection between the training and the work situation.

Dissatisfaction. Fill the gap where appropriate; remedy particular problems, such as pay or conditions.

Discipline. Disciplinary actions range from informal discussion – to increasingly formal procedures, and punishment – ultimately including dismissal.

Reorganising. This is where the problem has arisen through difficulties with the work materials, reporting relationships, or physical arrangements' being no longer adequately organized.

Management. Improve clarity in communicating the task, the monitoring systems, or the expertise of a particular manager.

Outside agencies. These are particularly appropriate when there are personal and family reasons.

The job. Transfer the individual to a more appropriate job or department; or redesign the job.

Peer pressure. When an individual's performance is very different from the average, those working alongside will recognise that it is inappropriate and may put pressure on the individual to change.

Source: D. Torrington and J. Weightman, *Action Management,* London, Institute of Personal Management, 1991.

Table 11 Check-list for handling a disciplinary matter

1. Gather all the relevant facts: promptly, before memories fade, take statements, collect documents, in serious cases consider suspension with pay while an investigation is conducted.

2. Be clear about the complaint: is action needed at this stage?

3. If so, decide whether the action should be:
   - advice and counselling
   - formal disciplinary action.

4. If formal action is required, arrange a disciplinary interview:
   - ensure that the individual is aware of the nature of the complaint and that the interview is a disciplinary one
   - tell the individual where and when the interview will take place and of a right to be accompanied
   - try to arrange for a second member of management to be present.

5. Start by introducing:
   - those present and the purpose of the interview
   - the nature of the complaint
   - the supporting evidence.

6. Allow the individual to state his/her case:
   - consider and question any explanations put forward.

7. If any new facts emerge:
   - decide whether further investigation is required
   - if it is, adjourn the interview and reconvene when the investigation is completed.

8. Except in very straightforward cases, call an adjournment before reaching a decision:
   - come to a clear view about the facts
   - if they are disputed, decide on the balance of probability what version of the facts is true.

9. Before deciding the penalty consider:
   - the gravity of the offence and whether the procedure gives guidance
   - the penalty applied in similar cases in the past
   - the individual's disciplinary record and general service
   - any mitigating circumstances
   - whether the proposed penalty is reasonable in all the circumstances.

10. Reconvene the disciplinary interview to:
    - clearly inform the individual of the decision and the penalty, if any
    - explain the right of appeal and how it operates
    - in the case of a warning, explain what improvement is expected, how long the warning will last and what the consequences of failure to improve may be.

11. Record the action taken:
    - if other than an oral warning, confirm the disciplinary action to the individual in writing
    - keep a simple record of the action taken for future reference.

12. Monitor the individual's performance:
    - disciplinary action should be followed up, with the object of encouraging improvement
    - monitor progress regularly and discuss it with the individual.

Source: ACAS, *Discipline at Work,* London, ACAS, 1987.

Discipline and dismissal

All the previous sections have been about disciplining in the sense of trying to change someone's performance; but at a certain point a manager may feel the process needs to be more formal. It is however advisable to keep records of what has happened from an early stage just in case things come to a formal procedure.

Most organisations, particularly the NHS, have procedures for discipline and dismissal. The personnel department and trade union representatives know them in detail. Many are based on the ACAS (Advisory Conciliation and Arbitration Service) code of practice; ACAS has an advisory booklet available on the subject. Table 11 shows the ACAS check-list for handling a disciplinary matter. If all this fails, and a decision about dismissal is considered, it is important that the correct procedure is adhered to, because the legislation on unfair dismissal is clear: you are advised to involve the personnel department and a senior manager as soon as possible.

Questions to ask yourself

Have I told a member of staff to change his or her behaviour?
Is this the second time?
Have I made a record of this?
To whom would I talk if I felt there was a problem member of staff?

And finally...

The 'red-hot stove' rule was originally advanced by the American industrial psychologist Douglas Macgregor, who likened effective discipline to touching a red-hot stove:

❏ The burn is immediate, so there is no question of cause and effect.

❏ There was warning: the stove was red hot, and you knew what would happen if you touched it.

❏ It is consistent: everyone touching the stove gets a burn.

❏ It is impersonal: you get a burn, not because of who you are but because of what you have done.

References

FLETCHER C. (1993) *Appraisal: Routes to improved performance.* London, Institute of Personnel Management.

GEORGE J. (1986) 'Appraisal in the public sector: dispensing with the big stick', *Personnel Management,* May, pp32–5.

KESSLER I. (1995) *Reward Systems in Human Resource Management: A critical text.* J. Storey (ed.). London, Routledge.

MACGREGOR D. (1960) *The Human Side of Enterprise.* New York, McGraw-Hill.

WEIGHTMAN J., BLANDAMER W. AND TORRINGTON D. (1991) 'Pay Structures and Negotiating Arrangements.' Report for the North Western Regional Health Authority.

CHAPTER 10

THE PEOPLE MANAGER AS SUSTAINER OF STAFF

Paul is in charge of the health education and promotion department. In the past year the department has moved from the purchasing authority to the community trust. He has six people working in his department with various skills, from professional health educationalist, photography, and publishing skills to event organisers. This year two local district health authorities (DHAs) and family health service authorities (FHSAs), including the one in which Paul is located, are amalgamating. A decision has been taken to merge Paul's department with the equivalent department in the neighbouring DHA/FHSA, which is established in one of the hospital healthcare trusts. Paul does not understand how this decision was taken, but his current concern is chiefly how to keep the staff going when they have already coped with a lot of change and feel that their jobs are vulnerable. Questions he asks himself are whether he should just put his head down and get on with working or lobby both inside and outside the department about the establishment of the new department, and what he can do to keep his staff going.

Not all of us have quite so many dramatic changes in a year as Paul and his colleagues, but most of us are having to deal with rapid changes. This chapter tries to answer the question, 'How can we help staff deal with change and keep things going when all around things are different?' People working in the health service are good at looking after the well-being of their patients, and often have quite exceptional skills at dealing with distress. But looking after the well-being of the staff is often left to others, or not done at all.

Usually the argument goes something like, 'Well, we must put the patients first.' We cannot expect a sustained period of effort from ourselves and others if we fail to ensure that staff are well. All of us can keep working like crazy for a few weeks, or indeed a few months if absolutely necessary, but this is not sustainable over a period of years – we will burn out. If we are investing in expensive selection and training of staff it is absurd to risk losing them because they are too exhausted to do their best work. Sustaining staff needs managing, and it is a line management role.

Handling people's responses to change

Innovations in organisational and technical aspects of health-care have meant that most people experience change in their work. To some, these changes mean excitement and the thrill of being 'part of the action'. For others, they feel like an ominous dismantling of the stable order of things. Although there is actually less change generally in society and industry in the UK now than at, say, the end of the nineteenth century, we all feel as if change is an everyday part of our lives. There are several kinds of change, which can be put into four broad types of experience.

- ❏ *Imposition*, when the initiative comes from someone else and we have to alter our ways of doing things to comply with outside requirements. This undermines our sense of being able to handle things, and we worry about the implications. New rules and laws are the obvious examples.

- ❏ *Adaptation*, when we have to change our behaviour or attitudes at the behest of others. This can be very difficult, and leads to people leaving or retiring. Examples are changes in attitude about race or gender, and taking on a business orientation rather than a public-service one.

- ❏ *Growth*, when we are responding to opportunities for developing competence, poise and achievement. An example is job changes.

- ❏ *Creativity*, when we are the instigator and therefore in control of the process. Examples would be introducing new standards at work, developing a new technique, or trying something to see whether it will work.

Most of us resist the first, are uncertain about the second, delighted with the third, and excited by the fourth kind of change. As a line manager you undoubtedly experience all of these and have to sustain your staff through periods of change. How can you best do so?

Questions to ask yourself

What sort of change have I experienced at work over the last 12 months?
Can I think of someone who responds well to change?
What about someone who responds badly to change?
What characteristics would I say describes each of them?

Managing change

The sequence for managing change goes something like this:

❑ Establish the project – what are you going to do?
❑ Set goals – what should be done, and by when?
❑ Identify a solution – how are we going to get there?
❑ Prepare for implementing – what resources do we need?
❑ Implement the project – how do we influence people and deal with the unexpected?
❑ Review progress – how are we doing?
❑ Maintain the project – are there any problems?

This is a useful check-list to prepare for change, but the important point is that, like trust and commitment, ownership of a project by the staff is built and develops over time. It comes through actually working to improve something. So it makes sense to give a firm push at the beginning of a project in order to get really started. Do not do so much planning that you never get to the action. It is also important to offer lots of help and support to your staff, which is better done after the initial planning. There is plenty of advice about how to manage change: see, for example, McCalman and Paton (1992). It is not my intention to deal in any detail with introducing change here.

There are several questions that you should ask when trying to persuade people to change, such as:

124

❑ What is in it for them? If they can see that the new behaviour, procedure, or technology will make their work more satisfying, they are more likely to be enthusiastic. If they cannot see any benefit, they are likely to resist.

❑ Have they had a say in the change? If people help to create a new scheme they are more committed to making it work. This should be a genuine opportunity to participate in the introduction, design, execution, and feedback of and from the new programme. If people are not involved at all, or the consultation is sham, their innovative and creative energies will often go into demonstrating just why something will *not* work.

❑ Is it clear what change is envisaged? We need a clear vision of what we are trying to achieve if we are to persuade others to get involved. It needs to be put into terms that others will understand; not everyone speaks in management terms!

Questions to ask yourself

What changes large or small have I experienced at work over the last three months?
Which of these were successfully achieved?
Does anything distinguish these from the more problematic?

When you want to introduce some new aspect to the work of your unit, try using the questions above.

Maintaining stability in a period of change

For a satisfactory life we all need a balance of novel experiences and ones that give us comfort or stability. How each of us wishes to balance these obviously varies from individual to individual, as does the interpretation of 'novelty' and 'comfort' – your comfort may be my novelty! The stimulation of novelty and change usually helps us to put effort into something. However, if the stimulation becomes too great we become less able to make a contribution (see Figure 6). It is at this point that stress is experienced, with all the associated feelings of increased tension and the possibility of failure.

Figure 6   Effect of stimulation and effort

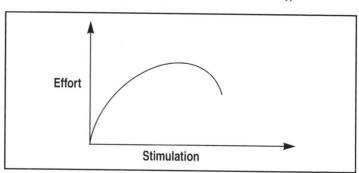

As long ago as 1970 Toffler recognised that we can cope with a lot of change, pressure, complexity, and confusion if at least *one* area of our lives is relatively stable (see Toffler 1970). We can rely on this stable part, and so risk change elsewhere. If we have nothing stable, everything becomes turmoil. He suggested that 'stability zones' were all-important to us, but that everyone had different ones. The main stability zones described by Toffler are:

❑ ideas – moral, religious, or political beliefs

❑ places – home, our town, the local pub, or place of work

❑ people – spouse, partner, parents, old friends with whom we share our life

❑ organisations – church, employer, or clubs that we belong to

❑ things and habits – routines, possessions, our cars.

We all need at least one of these to be secure. Working out where our stability zones are, and maintaining them, helps us to cope with stress in other areas.

Schein (1978) developed this idea of stability zones for the workplace. He coined the phrase 'career anchors' to suggest that there are distinct categories of stability zones at work that individuals evaluate themselves on. Each of us has one of the following as a most important feature of our working lives:

❑ managerial competence – seeking out opportunities to manage and take responsibility

❑ technical competence – enjoying the technical activity of nursing, physiotherapy, or medicine, for example

❑ security – job security, income, and pension

❑ creativity – important for those who want to build something of their own, such as a new process, theory, technique, or product

❑ autonomy and independence – where valuing freedom from constraints and having your own lifestyle are the most important things at work.

There are various other strategies for keeping one's balance when there is a period of rapid and unsettling change. In addition to the long-term strategy of trying to keep something stable, such as the stability zones or career anchors listed above, there are the smaller strategies such as trying to calm the pace at which you work by breathing slowly for a second or two. You might also try to remember that you do not have to deal with everything on your own: asking for help can bring new insights, companionship, and learning. Even just unloading your fears and frustration can make it easier to cope. But beware the danger of becoming an advice junkie!

Questions to ask yourself

What are my stability zones?
What are those of the people who work for me?
What about my career anchors?
Have any of the people who work for me got unreasonable career anchors?
To whom could I go for advice and succour with problems at work?

Coping with stress

The word 'stress' is very widely used these days and has come to mean a variety of things, so some definitions are required. Stress can refer to a stimulus for someone, eg 'The manager was putting a great deal of stress on the nurse and she resented it.' Stress can mean someone's response, eg 'The GP felt very stressed because of the number of patients who

127

had been discharged early from hospital.' Stress can also refer to the interaction of an individual and his or her environment, eg 'Working in the offices that faced onto the main interchange for the city's road system meant he felt stressed.'

There can be good and bad stress, over- and understress; when people talk about being 'stressed' they are usually referring to being overstressed with bad stress. The consequences of too much of this sort of stress are, in the long term, damaging to health and well-being. Research suggests that there is a link between the brain and the immune system, which means that depression and chronic stress arising from work and insomnia are often physically bad for us, because the activity of the immune cells goes up or down according to our different moods (see Mestel 1994). If this is so, then no wonder some illness is explained by the stress felt by individuals.

So what are the identifiable stressors at work, and what can be done about them? The overwhelming conclusion of behavioural studies of stress is that it is experienced in all occupations, but especially in manual work and particularly where there is routine repetitiveness and lack of autonomy (see Cooper and Earnshaw 1996). This lack of control over what we do and how we do it appears to be the most stressful work experience. Maybe this is one reason so many people in the NHS are claiming to be more stressed now: they feel more 'controlled' by financial considerations. Individual members of professional staff, particularly the medical staff, feel as if they have less personal autonomy than before, because managers have become more powerful.

Other areas to look for stressors at work include:

❑ the environment – eg, a culture of never saying you are overworked

❑ within oneself – eg, being nervous all the time

❑ interpersonal relationships – eg, thinking the other person is not trustworthy

❑ communication – eg, always insinuating things and never getting round to talking plainly

❑ workload – eg, five shifts can be more stressful than four shifts even if the hours are the same, because there is less time off work

❑ noise and physical conditions – eg, noisy machinery or conditions that are too hot or too cold are exhausting to work in, and this is especially stressful if precise judgements have to be made.

Intensive care units often have a high turnover of staff, which is associated with stressors such as grief, anxiety, guilt, exhaustion, overcommitment, and overstimulation.

There are various strategies for trying to cope with stress, other than the longer-term need to reduce the pressure. These are:

❑ emotional release – crying, drinking, praying
❑ physical release – diet, exercise, meditation, relaxation
❑ hobbies – distractions, holidays
❑ problem-solving – confrontation, assertion, action-planning
❑ personal and social support – family, friends, colleagues.

It is up to individuals to set up whichever of these is useful, but there are also well-established self-help groups in most localities, so I have not pursued the 'how to' here. If we are going to help our staff cope with their stress we clearly also need to start by coping with our own stress, using some of the above strategies.

Questions to ask yourself

What are the main causes of stress in my department?
Does everyone have something to call their own in their job?
Is there someone people can talk to in my department, either formally or informally, when they are feeling overwhelmed?
Do I encourage staff to develop life outside work?
Do I give them enough time to do so?
What about myself?

Managing time

One aspect of maintaining staff in periods of high demand is to help them to manage their time. It is also helpful to them and yourself if you manage your own time well so as to make as much time available as possible for 'having a chat'. One way to start doing this is to keep a simple activity diary for a few days, listing all the things you do as you go along. Then have a look at it and see how much you are doing to please others, and when and where you have a real choice about what to do (if anything). Another way is to use the analysis given in chapter 1 about sTAMp (see pages 9–10). Jobs vary enormously in the degree of choice available about what to do, but people vary enormously too in their interpretation of what is essential.

It is also worth making a list of all the demands that come to you over a couple of days in order to see just what decisions could be made about what to do (if anything). Most people are experiencing too many demands in their jobs at the moment. This means making choices: some things, clearly, have to be done, whereas some things can be left. The bulk, in the middle, are important things that need doing but not all of them can get done with the resources available. The normal advice is to prioritise these into 'must-dos' and 'hope-to-dos', with possibly some consultation with one's boss or co-workers. However, it is not always at all clear how one should do this. Frankly, if it is impossible to discriminate between equally important things that need doing, and you cannot do them all anyway, you might as well do the interesting ones and leave the others. You cannot do everything. Nowadays most of us are having to choose *not* to do things that appear worth doing (except of course those people without the opportunity of being in work at all). It is *learning to let go* of some of these that can lead to greater job satisfaction.

Questions to ask yourself

Have I actually got more choice than I think about what to do?
Have I carried on doing some things through habit even though they are no longer strictly necessary?
If so, is there some good reason for doing them – such as liking it?
Do I make too many demands on some individuals?

Ensuring health and safety

Through ignorance, carelessness, or neglect employers can endanger the health of those working in their organisation –

as well as that of patients, visitors, and local residents. An important aspect of managing people is to protect both the physical and psychological well-being of those whose lives the organisation affects. There is extensive legislation about health and safety, which gets ever more extensive as new inventions create fresh hazards not covered by existing laws. The basic protection for many years was a series of factory acts, mainly directed at protecting workers against long hours, and unsatisfactory space, ventilation, and heating.

A development of the factory acts came with the Control of Substances Hazardous to Health (COSHH) Regulations (1988), which comprise 19 different regulations and at least four codes of practice. The main features of all the regulations are:

- assessing the risks
- identifying what precautions are needed
- introducing measures to control or prevent the risk
- ensuring control measures are used
- making sure the procedures are followed
- getting equipment regularly maintained
- carrying out health surveillance
- informing the staff
- training the staff.

There is a risk that this system can become very bureaucratic and so use up a lot of resources rather than concentrating on the actual safety and well-being of people at work. However, there is a real responsibility for all managers to ensure that every member of staff, whether core or periphery, working in their section, knows of any hazardous substance or relevant health and safety procedure.

Much of this protection is now part of the EU's Social Chapter on the rights of workers, which the UK has not signed but which is being introduced by many multinational companies, and so is likely to become the norm for UK organisations.

Questions to ask yourself

Have we ensured that all the rotas stay within the permitted hours?
What are the hazardous substances and their associated procedures in our work?
Does everyone know about this (including students and placements)?

And finally...

In 1989 the Alliance and Leicester Building Society introduced term-time working for parents of school-age children (see Spencer 1990):

> Under the scheme, parents of children aged from five to fifteen may work during school terms only. Staff taking this option are given 10 weeks' unpaid leave every year to take during the school holidays, on top of which they are expected to take at least four weeks of their annual holiday entitlement during the school holidays. This minimum of 14 weeks' holiday amply covers the summer, Easter and Christmas breaks.

References

COOPER C. AND EARNSHAW J. (1996) *Stress and Employer Liability.* London, Institute of Personnel and Development.

MCCALMAN J. AND PATON R. A. (1992) *Change Management: a guide to effective implementation.* London, Paul Chapman.

MESTEL R. (1994) 'Let mind talk', *New Scientist* 23 July pp26–31.

SCHEIN E. (1978) *Career Dynamics: Matching individual and organisational needs.* Reading MA, Addison Wesley.

SPENCER L. (1990) 'Parent power', *Personnel Today.* April pp32-3.

TOFFLER A. (1970) *Future Shock.* London, Pan Books.

CHAPTER 11

THE PEOPLE MANAGER AS DEVELOPER AND TRAINER

Kate was head of the biochemistry department in a children's hospital. The department specialised in the detailed analysis of chemical disorders in young children, as well as the routine testing required by the hospital. In the past both she and her assistant attended several conferences a year, including one or two overseas trips. They also took junior staff with them when they had a particular expertise or interest in the subject under discussion. In this way they kept up to date with new advances and were seen to be contributing to the community of scientists. The children's hospital had become a healthcare trust, a result of which was that the budget for conferences and overseas travel was under constant attack.

How could Kate ensure that the department remained up to date? How was she to develop young scientists if there was no prospect of their attending conferences? Would she be able to attract first-class scientists if she could not give them a budget to meet other scientists? How were people going to build the network of contacts with fellow scientists if they met less frequently? Were there perhaps other ways of developing staff – such as seminars in the department, more systematic career development, job exchanges with other institutions, subscribing to journals with appropriate areas of expertise?

Training and developing staff are seen as an important part of managing people at work. However, finding the time and the money to pay for resources can be tricky. So why bother? There seems to be a consensus in the UK that training is a good thing. It is certainly felt to be at the heart of managing change. The government exhorts us to train through initiatives such as National Vocational Qualifications (NVQs) and Investors in People (IIP). Employers' organisations see training as the way to upgrade the skills of the workforce in order to take on new technologies and challenges from overseas. Trade unions see training and development as the way forward for members to keep jobs. All agree that encouraging staff to undertake training and development is one of the main tasks of managing people, whether this is the induction and training of a junior, the developing of an experienced member of staff, or the 'switching-on' of a jaded member of staff to adapt to changes sweeping through his or her organisation.

Deciding what skills to train and develop

The technical skills associated with systematic training are increasingly described in terms of: identifying the competencies required (see Chapter 8); measuring the competencies of the post-holders (see Chapter 9); identifying training needs and then developing those competencies that are less well-developed. Identifying training needs for the people whom one manages is done in a variety of ways. The most systematic is to compare the planned needs of the department with the assessed competencies of the people at present in the department, and work on the difference between these. Reality, fortunately, is never quite as mechanical as that!

Training needs are commonly identified in the following ways:

❑ at appraisal sessions, when the manager and the individual discuss what training would be appropriate over the next year to help improve and develop the individual's contribution and career prospects

❑ as a result of changes that the department is taking on, which may entail a training and development programme for the whole department

❑ at the instigation of the individual who wants to improve and develop his or her abilities either for current work or for long-term career purposes

❏ as part of the systematic progress of induction and initial training of new members of staff

❏ as part of a recovery programme after the identification of poor performance in an individual or group.

These training needs can be skills, knowledge, or understanding. Increasingly they are expressed in *competency* terms.

A competency is something that you can demonstrate: for example 'change gear while driving a car', or 'slice bread'. It is clear when the behaviour is successful. These behaviours can in turn be analysed into smaller steps when the overall competency is difficult to achieve. However, not all necessary work behaviours or competencies are easy to describe and analyse. Many of the most useful behaviours involve subtle application and experience to be effective. This means that many statements of and lists of competencies include knowledge, understanding, and personal attributes, as well as strictly behavioural descriptions.

Lists of competencies appropriate for a particular job, profession, or qualification can be drawn up by analysing and describing the behaviours and associated activities necessary to do specific aspects of the job. To this list is added the other behaviours likely to be required in the foreseeable future. Then appropriate assessment procedures can be devised for individuals to be assessed for selection, qualification, training, and development purposes. Training specialists have led the way in the use of these competency lists. Implicit in the whole competency approach is that the line manager is really involved in ensuring that the people they manage are given appropriate opportunities to develop.

With a list of the competencies required in a job and a measure of the competencies of the post-holder a comparison between the two is made and the areas for development or training needs identified. Then a programme of development can be agreed for the following period.

Questions to ask yourself

How do we identify what training we need in this department? Do we leave it up to individuals to volunteer, or is there another method?

What opportunities for development on the job do we encourage?

Are there any others in the department whom we could use for development purposes?

Have we started using a competency approach? Should we?

Deciding how to train and develop

Having decided what requires training and developing, the next question is how to go about it. A lot of the professional literature debates the niceties of different methods. Two useful books are those by Bee and Bee (1994) and Reid and Barrington (1996). Like most management decisions, those about training and development have to be made on the basis of the resources and opportunities available. It is useless planning a perfect but impracticable programme. This pragmatism should also be applied to what makes sense. There is absolutely no point in sending someone off on a long course if there is no prospect of his or her implementing the newly learnt skills when he or she comes back. Equally, there is no point trying to learn a new technique at work if the relevant equipment does not exist. There is also a cultural aspect to this: in more centralised organisations, staff are told what they need to learn and are given training to deliver this, whereas more self-managing organisations expect staff to identify their own learning priorities and find the resources available to achieve them.

A lot of different methods for training and development do exist, so I have included a brief description, in alphabetical order, of a number of the more common ways, along with some of the associated advantages and disadvantages. This is to allow you to think of something when faced with finding a training and development opportunity for one of your people.

Acting up

Acting up means doing a more senior job temporarily to cover for absence or vacancy (for example, maternity leave). It gives individuals the opportunity to broaden their experience and skill within a position of greater responsibility. The difficulty can be that returning to the original post after the acting-up period is difficult and needs sympathetic managing by the returning senior post-holder.

An example is the catering manager acting up for the hotel services director while she is off having a major operation.

Action learning

This involves the linking of a real, structured task with action inside the learning process using action learning sets. Action learning sets are groups of people who discuss the problems associated with the task using an identified facilitator. It can be difficult to keep the group on the task, as individuals develop, but it is a technique found particularly useful by senior staff, who enjoy being part of a group, when they can at times feel very isolated.

An example was a group of six personnel directors from two regional health authorities who came together to develop a personnel auditing form. The six originally met on a course but continued meeting infrequently with a facilitator over two years to complete the task.

Audiovisual presentations

These include slides, films and video. The technique is similar to a lecture in what it can achieve, but the advantage of video is that it can be stopped and started as required and be taken home to study at leisure.

An example are the numerous videos promoting new techniques and apparatus made by companies to market their products. Similarly, many journals now present their material on tape so that they can be listened to in the car on the way to work.

Case-studies

This is where a history of some event is given and trainees are invited to analyse the causes of a problem or indeed to find a solution. This provides an opportunity for a cool look at problems and for the exchange of ideas about possible solutions. However, trainees may not realise that the real world is not quite the same as the training session.

An example is the use made of case-studies for business development and taking on financial control. This might concern looking at various scenarios for a hospital trust, or case-studies of GP fundholders and the decisions they need to make about allocating financial resources. Another is the use of case-study presentations for the clinical development of doctors.

Coaching

This means improving the performance of someone who is already competent rather than establishing competency in the first place. It is usually done on a one-to-one basis, is set in the everyday working situation, and is a continuing activity. It is about gently nudging people to improve their performance, to develop their skills, and to increase their self-confidence so that they can take more responsibility for their own work and develop their career prospects. Most coaching is done by the senior person, but the subordinate position of the person coached is by no means a prerequisite. What is essential is that the coach should have the qualities of expertise, judgement, and experience that make it possible for the person coached to follow the guidance.

An example can be found in almost any contact between professionals: just think of some of the best interactions between clinical consultants and their juniors.

Delegation

Delegation is not just about giving jobs to do – it is about giving people the scope, responsibility, and authority to do it in their own way. It allows individuals to test their own ideas and to develop understanding and confidence. This is often called 'empowerment'. The more specific the instructions and terms of reference, the less learning results from the activity. With the assignment delegated, individuals start to work on their own. The decision about when to seek guidance and discussion on progress from the manager is also left in their own hands.

An example would be the director of estates handing over a portfolio of buildings to a junior who is given the autonomy, and budget, to decide how to maintain those buildings.

Discussion

This is where knowledge, ideas, and opinions on a subject are exchanged between trainer and trained. This is particularly suitable where the application is a matter of opinion, for changing attitudes, and for finding out how knowledge is going to be applied. The technique requires skill on the part of trainers because it can be difficult to keep discussion focused or useful.

One example was with the nursing and technical staff of an intensive care ward who, at the end of a day's training about performance appraisal, discussed with the trainer and senior staff how to go forward with an action plan.

Distance learning

This method involves individuals' using a range of printed, audiovisual, and other teaching materials outside the traditional course environment. It is a question of self-learning and requires high levels of personal discipline, and it can be difficult to sustain in isolation.

The Open University is probably the best-known example.

Empowerment

See 'Delegation' above.

Exercise

This is where trainees do a particular task in a particular way, to get a particular result. This is suitable when trainees need practice in following a specific procedure or formula to reach a required objective. The exercise must be realistic.

Most of us have had to do exercises to master the latest technology, such as PCs, faxes, answerphones, or video.

Group dynamics

Using this method, trainees are put in situations where their behaviour is examined. The task usually requires them to co-operate before they can achieve the goal. Observers collect information about how the trainees go about this and then give feedback to the group together and individually after the task is completed. The point is that trainees learn about the effect they have on others. This may appear rather threatening, and anxieties need to be resolved before the end of the session. This sort of development is very dependent on the quality of the trainer, and can be dangerous if adopted too casually. Usually the task is relatively remote from the realities of work.

The most common types of examples are outdoor activity centres on leadership for managers.

Job rotation

In job rotation individuals do different jobs within their section or organisation over a period of time. By setting up flexible working patterns within the organisation, individuals can be facilitated to broaden their experience and skills. The disadvantage can be the loss of highly specialised staff and their commitment to ensuring that things are right.

One example is the reorganisation of health visitors in some areas to take on a generic role, visiting the whole range of clients rather than specialising in particular types of work.

Learning contracts

These are usually agreed between individuals, their boss, and whoever is providing the learning experience. They specify what learning opportunities are expected, when these should occur, and what outcomes are expected. The aim is to ensure that everyone agrees; individuals are then expected to monitor their own performance against this contract. Contracts can also be used in conjunction with informal learning and to generate learning opportunities at work.

To give an example, second-year care students from a further education college had contracts agreed between the students, tutors, and the residential homes to which they were going on work-experience placements.

Learning opportunities

Many opportunities arise in the normal working environment that can be used for developing oneself or others. Look around and see what already exists before using time-consuming external opportunities. The difficulty is that these can be missed or that, by concentrating on the learning, the task itself is not carried out as efficiently.

Walking the floor is the classic way for managers to learn about the current concerns in their patch; this way they can also pick up on new ways of working. By using such information to ensure that individuals learn how to be more effective, useful development can take place – for example, observing that a nurse has found a way of getting a patient to accept his or her treatment and letting others see how it is done.

Lecture

A lecture is a talk given without much participation by the trainees. The method is suitable for large audiences, where the information to be got over can be worked out precisely in advance. There is little opportunity for feedback, so the lecturer may remain unaware that some in the audience have perhaps not got the point. Lectures require careful preparation and should ideally not be longer than 40 minutes. A lecture to doctors about a new medical finding at a conference is an obvious example of this technique.

On the job

With this method, trainees work in the real environment with support from a skilled person. This gives them real practice and it does not involve expensive new equipment. However, not all skilled people are skilled trainers. The essential ingredients are briefing, feedback, and support that help individuals to achieve the objectives in a structured way.

To take an example: a new business manager was in the office for two weeks before the old business manager moved on to a new job. This overlap meant a smoother handover of procedures and commitments, and provided an example of on-the-job training.

Programmed instruction

This can also be called computer-assisted learning (CAL). Trainees work at their own pace using a book or computer program that has a series of tasks and tests geared to teaching something systematically. It is suitable for learning logical skills and knowledge. However, it does not allow for discussion with others, which may be important when the application is debatable.

Examples are libraries with programs on how to use their services, or others on how to work out budgets or taxes, and business planning.

Projects

This is similar to an exercise (see above) but a project allows greater freedom for displaying initiative and creativity. Feedback may be given on a range of personal qualities as well as technical abilities. They need the full commitment and co-operation of the trainee, and specific terms of reference.

Management students at the Royal College of Nursing's Institute for Advanced Nurse Education have projects as part of several modules. These are expected to be work-based and practical, and are usually an opportunity for doing a more detailed study of something that needs to be done anyway, such as a business plan for a new development within the unit.

Role-play

In this method, people are asked to act the role they, or someone else, would play at work. It is particularly used in training for face-to-face situations, and is suitable for situations modelled on real-life when objective criticism would be useful. The difficulties are that people can be embarrassed, and the usefulness of the exercise is very dependent on the nature of the feedback given.

An example is the staff of the intensive care group mentioned above under 'Discussion' who practised interviewing one another using different techniques. They then role-played by conducting a mini-appraisal interview about one another's work during the previous week.

Secondment

This involves organising a placement in an alternative department or organisation for the achievement of a specific purpose. It is often used for management and professional development. The individual may, of course, choose not to come back!

A common example for doctors is going on secondment to a particular hospital, often abroad, to learn specific techniques and standards. For example, an orthopaedic surgeon went to the Mayo clinic in the USA for three months just before taking up a consultant post in the UK.

Simulation

This training method involves the use of situations modelled on real-life and real equipment. It gives people experience before they encounter the real thing and can be used for initial training, updating, keeping in practice, or introducing new techniques. The expense of creating a realistic mock-up is justified only when practising on the real thing is impossible or when a mistake would be catastrophic. The increasing sophistication of computer graphics have enabled all sorts of simulations and 'virtual reality' to be created for workplace training and development.

Obvious examples are the cadavers used for medical students and surgeons as a traditional sort of simulation. An example of computer simulation is a program for training ambulance service control-room staff in the use of a new system for contacting ambulances.

Skill instruction

Here the trainee is told how to do it, shown how to do it, and then does it under supervision. This is suitable for putting across skills, as long as the task is broken into suitable parts. What is considered 'suitable' varies with the task and the person receiving the training. Breaking things down into small steps is not suitable for all skills, because some are better learnt as a whole.

Any mechanical skill would be a good example here, such as learning how to put up a drip, how to service the machines or stripping down the airconditioning in the theatres.

143

Talk

A talk allows trainees to participate by asking questions or by having questions asked of them. It is useful for getting over a new way of looking at things that involve abstraction. It is appropriate for up to 20 people, but can only be used when people are willing to participate.

Examples are when ideas about management or the future are being explored. Management consultants usually report their findings to the board by giving a presentation, after which individuals ask questions and test their grasp of the findings.

Questions to ask yourself

Which of the above methods would be best suited to short-term (ie less than six months) training and development?
Which would be better suited to long-term goals?
Which are appropriate for introducing new working practices that everyone needs to adopt?
Which require a degree of self-confidence and motivation?
Which would I find easy to resource, and which require major expenditure?

Evaluating training

If organisations and people are to spend time, effort and money on training and development it is important to evaluate whether it has really been useful. 'Validation' describes the process of seeing whether the training and development have achieved their objectives, whereas 'evaluation' is the process of ascertaining whether the training has affected the performance of the job. It may be that the outward-bound leadership course has met all the objectives – validation – but we cannot see any change in performance at work – evaluation. Evaluation is much more difficult because of the problems of deciding, defining, and measuring performance or competency. Hamblin (1974) suggest five levels at which evaluation may take place:

❑ reaction – trainees give their personal view and impressions of the experience

144

- learning – the amount of learning is measured
- job behaviour – work behaviour is looked at six to nine months later to see if it has changed
- organisation – productivity, time taken to do things, absenteeism, turnover, and labour costs are examined to see if there is a difference after the training
- ultimate level – the effect on profitability and growth over a period of years.

At a line-management level you probably do not want to get involved in elaborate evaluation of any training you use, because the cost-effectiveness of doing so would not be justified. However, it is worth having some simple sort of evaluation, if only at the level of asking 'Do we think this has been useful?' or 'Would we do this again?'

Questions to ask yourself

Which sort of evaluation do we use?
Would it be cost-effective to carry out more?

Encouraging lifelong learning or personal development

Increasingly organisations, professional bodies, and the government are emphasising the need for individuals to develop and learn throughout their lives so that they can cope with the increasing speed of change. The argument goes like this: the more learning that is undertaken, the easier it becomes, and the more confident the individual will have, to face changes and move from one employer to another (an increasingly likely situation, now that lifetime employment is rare). This emphasis on lifetime personal development is enshrined in two formal initiatives:

- *Continuous Professional Development (CPD).* Many professional bodies (although not all) are emphasising CPD and expect their members to fulfil a minimum training requirement every year to maintain membership. Some of this CPD experience is credit-bearing, leading to further qualifications and higher ranking within the profession.

❏ *Investors in People (IIP)*. This is a government-backed initiative to encourage organisations to train and develop their staff. When suitable systems of identifying training and development needs and then carrying out the required programmes of training and development take place, organisations are entitled to a certificate as 'investors in people'. This has proved popular with organisations in both the private and public sectors.

There is a parallel emphasis on the learning organisation, which is able to encourage individuals to take on change and new tasks by a process of continuous learning.

Another aspect of encouraging lifetime personal development concerns the management of individual careers. Managers have to learn to manage talent, which includes developing staff so that they build careers to suit themselves. This is increasingly important if Kanter's (1989) comments are true about security of employment coming from being employable rather than from being employed by a particular employer. All of us need opportunities to develop skills and a reputation. This involves ensuring that people get a variety of opportunities and experiences. As Handy (1989: 104) puts it, managers have to be:

> teacher, counsellor and friend, as much or more than he or she is commander, inspector and judge.

My colleague Valmai Bowden, looking at the careers of bench scientists, has pointed out that this nurturing of people's careers can be compared to parenting. Some managers are very strict and dogmatic ('Do like me!') whereas others are more facilitating and encourage self-direction and assessment. Workers who are lucky enough to have good 'parenting' from their managers are likely to develop into the confident, learning, self-developing individuals who should go on to have rewarding careers. Those who feel ignored and rejected can become embittered. Maybe this facilitating of people's careers is at the heart of the relationship between managers and the managed in the new empowered climate.

146

Questions to ask yourself

In what ways do I encourage my staff to develop careers appropriate to each of them?

Do I expect them to want the same things that I do?

Do I encourage learning in all the staff, including the established members?

And finally...

Try justifying a skiing holiday in terms of the opportunities it gives for teambuilding and developing skills in a group of managers.

References

BEE F. AND BEE R. (1994) *Training Needs Analysis and Evaluation.* London, Institute of Personnel and Development.

HAMBLIN A. (1974) *Evaluation and Control of Training,* London, McGraw-Hill.

HANDY C. (1989) *The Age of Unreason.* London, Business Books.

KANTER R. M. (1989) *When Giants Learn to Dance.* London, Simon & Schuster.

REID M. A. AND BARRINGTON H. (1996) *Training Intervention: Managing Employee Development.* 6th edn, London, Institute of Personnel and Development.

CHAPTER 12

THE PEOPLE MANAGER AS COMMUNICATOR

Susan is a physiotherapist working in the small community hospital of a market town. The hospital is right in the centre of town, literally surrounded by the market on market days. Most of Susan's time is taken up seeing patients (including several elderly people) whom she has got to know well over the 10 years she has been in her present job. Susan has six part-time colleagues in her department. Two of them have come separately to Susan to say that they refuse to work with each other again, and can she please ensure that they are never on the same rota in future? What should Susan do?

It is certainly not her intention to comply with their request, as she feels this is unprofessional – and in any case it would reduce her choices for cover and holidays. What sort of communication does she need to have with each of the members of staff? What sort of communication does she need to encourage them to have with each other? Should anyone else be involved? Fortunately, Susan was ready for this sort of encounter, because she had been the professional association representative for years and was also an experienced local authority councillor, both of which facts meant she had had lots of practice at formal communication with colleagues.

Most of the communication that you will need to use as a health worker and as a manager will be face to face with a patient, a member of your staff, or a small group. You may also need to have face-to-face discussions with other people within and without the organisation. Professionally, you may well have developed very good communication skills with patients, but perhaps you are worried about some of the more formal or critical face-to-face encounters in your management role. Effectiveness in any of these situations is one of the keys to successful management performance. Communicating is at the heart of getting things done. It can mean a person persuaded to follow a new administrative procedure. It may mean explaining and justifying the logic of the new infection control plan. A problem eased, or enthusiasm engendered in someone else, are both examples of good communication. There are also briefing sessions and everyday conversations for social contact and stimulation that maintain smooth, co-operative relations. Each requires some variation of the manager's personal style of communication – difficulties can arise if these varying demands are not understood.

Improving communication

Communication is a two-way process, complete only when the message is received and understood, even if the understanding is not exactly what was intended. Both the sender and the receiver of a message have an active part to play. This reciprocal process is sometimes described as the *communications model* or *speech chain,* and systems or information theory terms are used to describe it. For effective communication to take place, each of the following six stages should be operating well: encoding, transmitting, the environment, receiving, decoding, and feedback (see Figure 7). Problems of communication can occur at any or all of these different phases in the chain. If we consistently have problems communicating with one another, it can be worthwhile sitting down and analysing where in this chain we think the problem may lie.

To be effective communicators we should consider not only our own performance but also that of the people we are trying to communicate with, and the likely effect upon them of what we are saying and how we are saying it. Understanding other people is difficult because we all have a different set of operating assumptions (see Chapter 5 for discussion of individual differences), according to which we conduct our lives. If we do not recognise this diversity, communication becomes at best awkward and at worst non-existent.

149

Figure 7 The basic communications model or speech chain

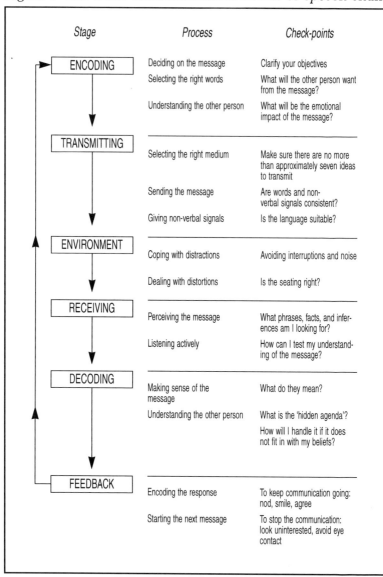

Factors other than those involved in direct communication can also affect the outcome of a conversation or meeting. Physical things such as noise and temperature are obvious factors. The position of the furniture can also play a part: seating a group so that everyone can see each other increases interaction – think of how seminars and training sessions in which you sit in a circle vary from those in which you sit in rows. Having a table between participants increases formality but gives them (quite literally) something to hold on to if it is a tense situation. Interruptions from the telephone or keeping an 'open door' can disrupt communication.

Difficulties in communication may occur because:

- the purpose of the communication is unclear
- there are problems in sending the message
- there are problems in receiving the message
- outside physical factors interfere.

Where effective communication is critical, each stage needs to be considered so as to pre-empt any problems.

Questions to ask yourself

What differences ought I to expect in the communication chain for the following sorts of communication:
- communicating to achieve or obtain something
- communicating to get someone to behave differently
- communicating to find out something
- communicating my feelings
- communicating to enjoy companionship
- communicating to sort out a problem
- communicating for interest
- communicating because the situation demands it?

Using transactional analysis

Another approach to analysing communication difficulties has been the psychiatric and therapeutic models of counselling. One that has enjoyed much popularity is a simple device originated by Berne (1966), who suggests that we

151

interact with one another by means of behaviours that can be described as *parent, adult* or *child*. 'Parent' behaviour is one of authority and superiority; a person behaving in this way is typically dominant and even likely to scold. This is the ego state, in which all our value judgements are stored, and also the state of a person every time he or she behaves like a parent. The 'child' state contains all the unpredictability of tantrum and charm, obedience and defiance, tears and laughter, sulks and joy. The parent acts in the way he or she was taught; the child acts in the way he or she feels, impulsive and uncensored. Someone in the 'adult' state is objective and rational, analysing situations as realistically as possible, processing information, estimating probabilities, and making decisions. This state is not prejudiced by the values of the parent, or by the natural urges of the child. These labels have nothing to do with age; nor do we fit into only one of these categories. All of us have all three states, and spend each day moving from one to the other.

We therefore have all three sorts of behaviour, and can bring any one of them into play when we communicate. This means that when we communicate with one another, all combinations are possible. The most frequent types of transaction are: complementary, crossed, and ulterior (see Figure 8).

❑ A *complementary* transaction is an appropriate and expected one, and follows the natural order of relationships.

❑ *Crossed* transactions are those when an opening statement elicits an inappropriate response.

❑ *Ulterior* transactions are more complex, because they always involve more than two ego states. The most common occurs when the real message is disguised under an explicit and more socially acceptable one.

In most situations at work the ideal transaction is adult–adult, but any complementary transaction is better than any crossed one. If two people are both in 'child mode' and start shouting at each other, they are not going to resolve their differences; but at least they will probably cope better than if one of them starts being a parent! You might find it useful

Figure 8 Transactions

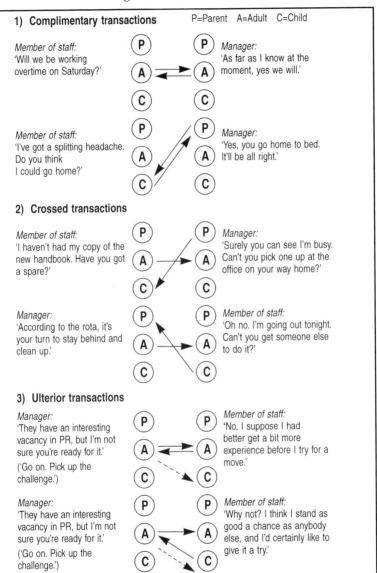

1) Complimentary transactions   P=Parent A=Adult C=Child

Member of staff:
'Will we be working
overtime on Saturday?'

Manager:
'As far as I know at the
moment, yes we will.'

Member of staff:
'I've got a splitting headache.
Do you think
I could go home?'

Manager:
'Yes, you go home to bed.
It'll be all right.'

2) Crossed transactions

Member of staff:
'I haven't had my copy of the
new handbook. Have you got
a spare?'

Manager:
'Surely you can see I'm busy.
Can't you pick one up at the
office on your way home?'

Manager:
'According to the rota, it's
your turn to stay behind and
clean up.'

Member of staff:
'Oh no. I'm going out tonight.
Can't you get someone else
to do it?'

3) Ulterior transactions

Manager:
'They have an interesting
vacancy in PR, but I'm not
sure you're ready for it.'
('Go on. Pick up the
challenge.')

Member of staff:
'No, I suppose I had
better get a bit more
experience before I try for a
move.'

Manager:
'They have an interesting
vacancy in PR, but I'm not
sure you're ready for it.'
('Go on. Pick up the
challenge.')

Member of staff:
'Why not? I think I stand as
good a chance as anybody
else, and I'd certainly like to
give it a try.'

to use this transactional analysis format when communication is getting nowhere, feels too emotional, or when the relationship is somehow awkward. By clarifying how you are tripping each other up you might stand more chance of understanding how to change the way you respond.

Questions to ask yourself

Next time you find yourself having an awkward conversation with someone, analyse it afterwards, using Berne's model, and see if it makes any more sense.

Can I think of colleagues who frequently behave in parent, child, or adult mode?

Do I have particular difficulties with any of these?

Conducting formal interviews

One area that concerns many professionals when they start managing staff is the business of conducting formal interviews, whether for appraisal, recruitment, or disciplinary reasons. Usually the content is fairly well known, but the process of interviewing is less familiar. The important thing to remember is that you have to 'conduct' the formal interview. That means taking responsibility for how it is structured and when it will start and finish. The person interviewed will expect you to do so and will feel let down if nothing happens in the interview. This is different from a counselling interview, in which there is a joint problem-solving approach, although even here you as the manager are expected to conduct the process. So you need to prepare what you want out of the interview. What is its purpose? What needs to be covered? You may well be used to doing this with your patients but, usually, a formal interview with a member of staff lasts longer than the time allowed with patients, so you need to think about how to conduct the flow of the conversation. Table 12 is a suggested format of questions for making the interview flow appropriately.

Table 12   Interviewing

1   Getting Started

Establish rapport, so that participants get used to each other's tone, volume and personality. Methods include: small talk, friendly manner, calm attention and explaining what is going to happen.

2   Keeping it going

Maintain rapport and keep the communication to the agenda. Methods include: showing interest, giving verbal and non-verbal signals of agreement, making encouraging noises but keeping silent at times when other people are considering points. It may sometimes be necessary to bring suppressed feelings into the open by asking a question like 'Is there something on your mind ...?'

3   Questions

There are different types of question according to what you want to do:

Type	Purpose	Example
Closed	To seek precise information	'What is your name?'
Open	To get opinions developed	'How do you do that?'
Direct	To insist on a reply	'Why did you do that?'
Indirect	An oblique approach to a difficult matter	'What were they like?'
Probe	To obtain information that is being withheld; one way is to exaggerate	'You weren't in prison, were you?'
Proposing	To put forward an idea	'Shall we do as Tom suggests?'
Rhetorical	To forbid a reply	'We're not afraid of the competition, are we?'

4   Stopping

❑ Slow the general rate of talking by slipping one or two closed questions into the conversation and eliminating encouraging gestures.
❑ Gather your papers together and say something to indicate closing, such as 'Well, I think we have covered the ground ...'
❑ Explain the next step, such as who does what.
❑ Stand up.

Source: D. Torrington and J. Weightman, *Action Management,* London, Institute of Personnel Management, 1991.

Questions to ask yourself

Who wants what from this interview?
Are there any other constraints or choices available to us?
Do we need to take a decision now?
What is the follow-up to the interview?
Try using the sequence in Table 12.

Communicating with the whole department, section, or team

Sometimes we need to communicate with the whole work group. This might be in order to ensure that everyone knows about, and is using a particular method, standard, or procedure; that is, some sort of *regulation* needs to be communicated. It might be a matter of seeking to change some aspect of how we work, such as how can we reduce waste, introduce some new software on the PCs, or change the appointment system for patients; that is, some sort of *innovation* is to be communicated. A third sort of communication occurs when we try to raise morale and develop a feeling of identity within the group through jokes or by planning an outing; that is, communicating *integration*. We might also want to get over factual *information* that people need in order to get on with their work.

Each of these four main types of communication – regulation, innovation, integration, and information – can be achieved through speaking with people, writing to them, or including a non-verbal aspect to the communication. For most purposes we probably make an automatic choice as to the appropriate way to communicate particular messages. There is certainly local custom and practice about the 'way we say things round here'. However, it is sometimes worth trying a different way, particularly when communication does not seem to be quite as effective as you would like. Table 13 may give you some suggestions. I have just given examples in this table, because it is surprising how very different organisations are in the way they communicate these four fundamental aspects of organisational life.

156

Table 13   Communicating with the whole work group

Regulation

Speaking	Departmental meetings	
	Directions and requests	
	Catching everyone at break-times and change of shift	
Writing	Agenda for meeting	
	Job descriptions	
	Performance standards	
	Memos	
	E-mail	
Non-verbal	Gesture	
	Pauses and silences	

Innovation

Speaking	Problem-solving meetings	
	Conversations	
	Team briefings	
	Brainstorming	
Writing	Reports on visits and courses	
	Suggestions schemes	
	E-mail	
	Journals	
Non-verbal	Seating arrangements	
	Laughter	

Integration

Speaking	Saying hello	
	Coffee breaks	
	Ritual of acknowledging birthdays	
Writing	Letters of congratulation on passing courses	
	House-style stationery	
	E-mail	
	Report forms in house style	
Non-verbal	Eye contact in the corridor	
	State of staff room	
	Staff socials	

Information

Speaking	Training sessions	
	Mass meeting	
	Change over time for shifts	
Writing	Memos	
	Notice board	
	E-mail	
	Handbooks	
	Bulletins and newsletters	
Non-verbal	Demonstrate what needs doing	
	Having an example	

Questions to ask yourself

Using Table 13 as a template, see if you can find examples of each category at work.
Were any of the categories particularly easy to find?
Were any particularly difficult?
How do I communicate integration?
Compare my experience with someone in another part of the same organisation or another organisation altogether. What are the main differences?

For which of the following would you use verbal, written, or non-verbal methods, or a combination of them, to communicate:

❑   changed safety regulations
❑   a new procedure for claiming travel expenses
❑   proposals for merging two departments
❑   a change to holiday arrangements
❑   information regarding a particular patient and their family situation?

Communicating effectively in meetings

Many managers spend a lot of time attending, and complaining about, meetings. The usual question is, 'What is the point of this meeting?' Meetings have both overt and covert reasons for taking place. Some of these reasons are given below.

Overt reasons for meetings

❑   *Making decisions.* The meeting may be the focus of a decision-making process, with all the appropriate people present. Or, as often happens, prior discussions have arrived at the decisions and the meeting merely ratifies them.

❑   *Making recommendations.* Those assembled have to agree whether to recommend something – and, if they do want to recommend it, to whom. This might only be a subsidiary meeting to recommend a motion to a more senior meeting at which the real decision will take place.

❑   *Training newcomers to the group.* It is often through attending meetings that managers learn about the wider implications of the work of their unit and the issues facing the organisation as a whole. It is also a source of learning about the politics and power-play within the organisation.

❏ *Analysis and report.* Here, the purpose of the meeting is to organise material for another group. This is particularly the function of working parties.

❏ *Information.* In this instance people have met to exchange and ask for information, something that usually takes place under the 'any other business' or 'matters arising' sections of formal meetings.

Covert reasons for meetings

❏ *Cohesion.* People may be encouraged to feel part of the whole by chatting beforehand, catching someone's eye, or joking. Some regular meetings try to engender this 'club-biness' by having regular breakfast meetings of the management team or an occasional 'away day' in a hotel.

❏ *Catharsis.* Sometimes it is useful to give vent to anger even when nothing can be done. At least people feel they 'have had their say'.

❏ *Manipulation.* This occurs when a particular decision or action is desired and the meeting is manoeuvred into agreeing to this as if it was their own decision and is usually done by the more senior staff.

Questions to ask yourself

This is a check-list developed to consider the arrangements for regular meetings (Torrington and Weightman 1989). It was designed to assist in running them effectively so that the necessary communication and decision-making can take place. The list of questions might also help when a regular meeting feels wrong, because this usually means something on the list below is not clear or agreed on. There are no right answers: it is just a list for you to consider.

Who should attend the meeting:

❏   a large group to represent wide interests

❏   a small group to make discussion easier and more productive

❏ representatives of each layer in the hierarchy
❏ a variety of personalities to ensure a lively discussion
❏ only those with expertise in this area?

The brief or terms of reference of the meeting:
❏ Does this meeting have the power to take a decision?
❏ Can this meeting make a recommendation?
❏ How wide can the discussion usefully range?
❏ Has a decision relating to this topic already been made that cannot be changed?
❏ Are there some conclusions that would be unacceptable? If so, to whom?

The agenda:
❏ What do we need to consider, and in what order?
❏ Is there too much to cope with?
❏ Who can add items to the agenda?
❏ Will 'matters arising' and 'any other business' take up a lot of time?

The physical location and arrangements:
❏ Does everyone know which room we shall meet in, and is it the right size?
❏ Is the furniture arranged so that everyone can see every one else and make eye contact with them?
❏ Is it appropriate to have coffee served? Has it been arranged?
❏ Is the room noisy or cold?
❏ Are there likely to be interruptions?

Stimulating and controlling contributions:
❏ Who has something to say?
❏ How can I get them to say it?
❏ How can I keep the long-winded brief?
❏ When should I nudge the meeting towards a decision or the next item?

Minutes or report of the meeting:
❏ Who writes these?
❏ Is it important to describe the discussion and issues, or just make a list of actions and who is responsible for them?
❏ Who gets a copy?
❏ What will be the effect of the minutes on those who attended (and those who did not)?

❏   Whom are we trying to influence with these minutes, and in what way?

Implementation of proposals:
❏   Who has agreed to do what?
❏   How can we help one another to get on with it?
❏   Whom else can we involve?
❏   How can we monitor the implementation?
❏   Do we need a review date?
❏   What can I do to get things moving?

And finally...

Consider the following sayings:

'The audience were on the edge of their seats.'

'She gave me the cold shoulder.'

'He remained poker-faced throughout.'

'Speech is silver; silence is golden.'

'She is down in the mouth today.'

'He is all ears.'

'She is a stuck-up person.'

'He is on his high horse.'

'Her face lit up...'

What do these suggest to you about effective and non-verbal communication?

References

BERNE E. (1966) *Games People Play*. London, André Deutsch.

TORRINGTON D. AND WEIGHTMAN J. (1989) *Management and Organisation in Secondary Schools: A training handbook*. Oxford, Blackwell.

INDEX